Alzheimer's Disease and the Eye

Jeffrey N. Weiss

Alzheimer's Disease and the Eye

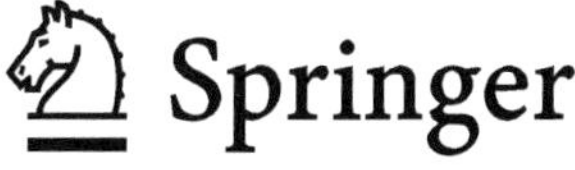 Springer

Jeffrey N. Weiss
Parkland, FL, USA

ISBN 978-3-031-58813-6   ISBN 978-3-031-58811-2   (eBook)
https://doi.org/10.1007/978-3-031-58811-2

This Springer imprint is published by the registered company Springer Nature Switzerland AG
The registered company address is: Gewerbestrasse 11, 6330 Cham, Switzerland

If disposing of this product, please recycle the paper.

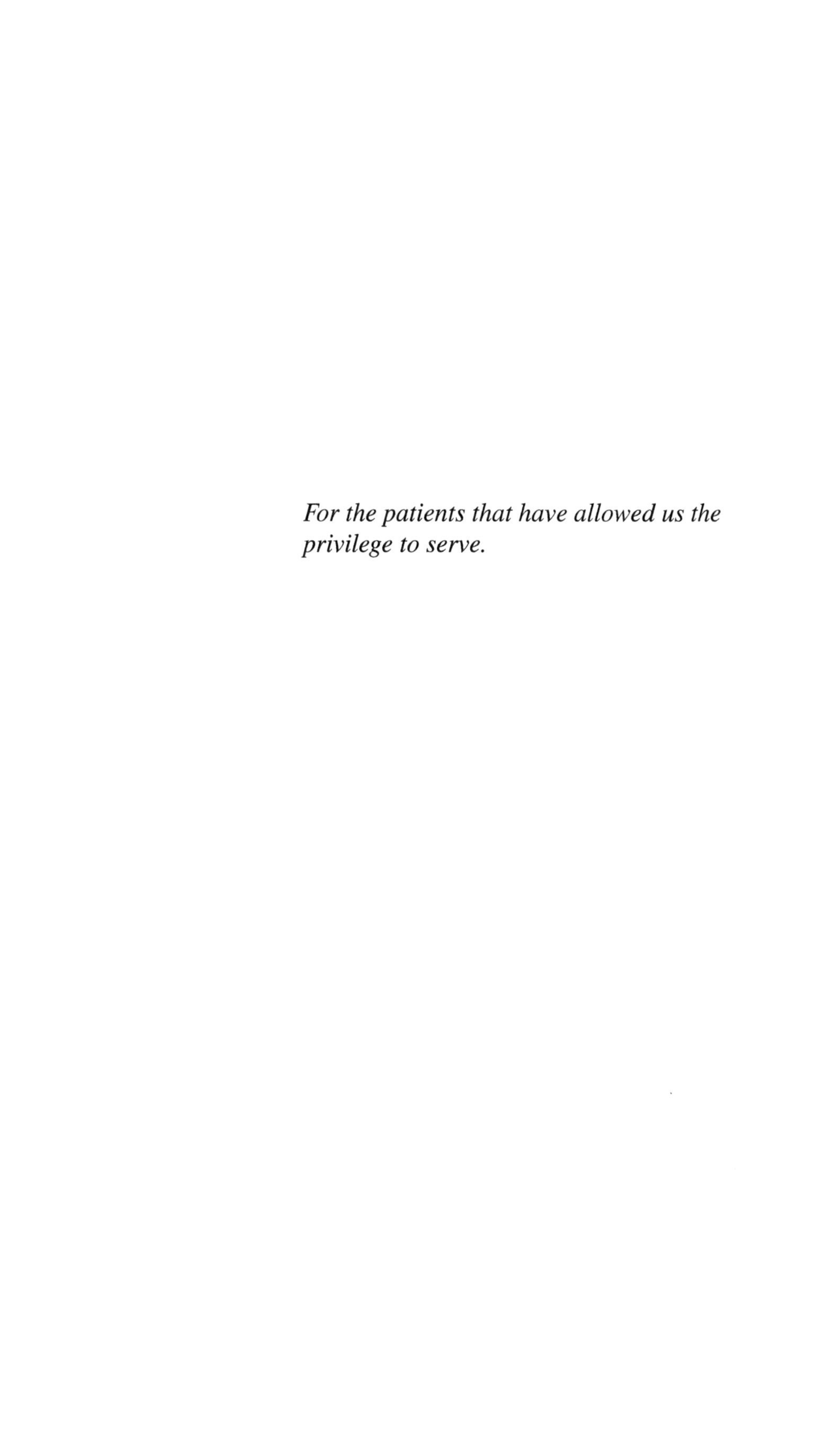

For the patients that have allowed us the privilege to serve.

Preface

This book is a compendium of the worldwide studies of Alzheimer's disease utilizing the eye as a biomarker, or as a treatment method, that are registered with the United States National Institutes of Health website, clinicaltrials.gov. Clinicaltrials. gov is the largest listing of research studies in the world. The presented information is accurate as of October, 2023. I have divided the studies into Recruiting, Not Yet Recruiting, Active, Not Recruiting, and Enrolling By Invitation.

In order to produce an accurate, consistent, and easy-to-read format, I corrected the mischaracterization of studies by only including those that truly belonged within each category, and corrected spelling and grammar, without changing the spirit or intentions of the submitters. The Study Title is provided, as is the Country of Origin and the Clinical Trial Number in order to make it easier for the reader to locate the study and obtain further information.

From a conceptual standpoint, early diagnosis of a clinical condition offers the potential of a better outcome. Earlier intervention is better than late intervention when the die may already be cast and progression to a negative end result can no longer be prevented.

What is meant by "early diagnosis?" How early is early? The temporal determination is related to the ability to affect the outcome. Would most people truly wish to know that in 10 years they will develop Alzheimer's disease, if there was no way to prevent it? Understandably, some might say "yes" as that knowledge would cause them to lead a healthier lifestyle, to refrain from tobacco and alcohol usage, and to exercise more. All worthy goals. But what if it also led to the person quitting their job, getting divorced, and engaging in risky activities because they felt that their fate was already sealed? And if, 10 years later, in the absence of any preventative treatment, they didn't develop the condition? Was the test just incorrect, did a change in lifestyle prevent the negative outcome, or were they just lucky? Of course, during the 10-year period a new treatment may be discovered that precludes the prior negative assured outcome.

I think most people would agree that unless there is a meaningful, successful treatment for an early diagnosis, there is no point in knowing many years in advance of the inevitable when there is little you can do to change the outcome. Lead your life and let what may come.

New drug development is costly and time consuming. If, through the use of biomarkers, study durations and research costs decrease, there is a greater possibility of a new and effective drug to treat this devastating disease. The eye offers the possibility of early diagnosis and of treatment.

I hope that by providing this reference, the field of ocular research in Alzheimer's disease will be advanced.

Parkland, FL, USA

Jeffrey N. Weiss

Contents

Chapter 1
Introduction

Alzheimer's Disease

Alzheimer's disease is a progressive, degenerative brain disorder leading to death. Early-onset Alzheimer's disease (ages 30–65) is strongly related to hereditary and genetics. Late-onset Alzheimer's (age 65 and older) is the leading cause of dementia, affecting more than 5 million Americans. While associated with advancing age, there is no evidence that the disease is caused by the aging process. While particular genes may increase susceptibility to late-onset Alzheimer's, researchers are studying the effect of genetic, environmental, dietary, infectious agents, and metabolic abnormalities that may lead to disease's development.

Unfortunately, at the present time, there is no simple clinical test to diagnose this condition. Posthumously, neuritic plaques composed of amyloid protein and/or neurofibrillary tangles of tau protein are found. The average life expectancy following the diagnosis is 5–10 years. There is no successful treatment, drugs may improve symptoms in some cases.

In the last decade, more than 500 drug studies have failed to find a truly successful treatment for this condition. In the absence of a definitive quantitative endpoint, most studies have been terminated after 2 years, yet 5–10 years would have been required to determine a meaningful clinical effect.

The eye is the only place in the body where an artery, vein, and nerve can be directly visualized. The nerve fiber layer of the retina is an outgrowth of the brain. Retinal thinning is observed by noninvasive Ocular Coherence Tomography testing in patients diagnosed with Alzheimer's disease. It is apparent that a much earlier molecular effect would lead to an imaging change.

If an early, noninvasive, and cost-effective method is discovered to diagnose "early" Alzheimer's disease, then (a) pharmaceutical companies may shorten

J. N. Weiss, *Alzheimer's Disease and the Eye*, https://doi.org/10.1007/978-3-031-58811-2_1

clinical studies, at lower research costs, leading to the development of new, effective drugs, and (b) physicians may identify patients with early disease, and prescribe the new drugs.

Rates of Dementia

Worldwide, Alzheimer's disease affects 5–8% of the general population greater than 60 years of age, or 50 million people at the present time. Sixty percent of the affected patients are in low- to middle-income countries. There are 10 million new cases per year; 82 million affected patients are projected in 2030, and 152 million in 2050.

Alzheimer's disease represents 60–70% of dementia cases, though there may be an indistinct boundary between the different types, and a patient may exhibit mixed dementia.

In 2015, the global cost of care was $818 billion US dollars, or 1.1% of the global GDP (0.2% in low- to middle-income nations to 1.4% in high-income countries).

In the United States, more than 5 million Americans are living with Alzheimer's dementia; 10% of people are older than 65 years of age and two-thirds of the patients are women. African-Americans are twice as likely as Caucasians to have Alzheimer's disease. Hispanics are 1.5× as likely as Caucasians to develop Alzheimer's. By 2050, in people age 65 and older—13.8 million of Americans will be diagnosed with Alzheimer's disease.

From 2000 to 2018 deaths from Alzheimer's increased 146%, while deaths from cardiac disease decreased by 7.8%. Sixty-one percent of 70-year-olds with Alzheimer's will die by age 80, while only 30% of 70-year-olds without Alzheimer's will die by age 80.

Seventy percent of the cost of caring for a family member with Alzheimer's is borne by families.

Twice as many Alzheimer's caregivers (compared to non-Alzheimer caregivers) report emotional, financial, and physical difficulties.

2020 US cost 305 billion (206 billion paid by Medicare/Medicaid)
2050 projected cost 1.1 trillion (in 2020 dollars)

The NIH website, www.clinicaltrials.gov, lists 470,354 research studies in the United States and in 222 other countries.

Alzheimer's disease—	2870 studies worldwide, 1503 US studies (accessed 7/14/22)
	3243 studies worldwide, 1701 US studies (accessed 10/24/23)

Biomarkers play increasingly informative roles in Alzheimer's disease trials.

Biomarkers/Clinical Endpoints

A biological marker, or biomarker, is an objective measurable indicator of a biological state, including, normal and pathologic biologic conditions, and the response to therapeutic interventions. Biomarkers are biologic molecules found in tissue, blood, or other bodily fluids. A biomarker must have validity or evaluation, that is, its effectiveness as a relevant endpoint. The biomarker must also demonstrate clinical relevance, does it provide clinically relevant information? Biomarkers are objective and quantifiable, but unlike a clinical endpoint, may not reflect the patient's well-being from their standpoint. Examples include chemistry tests, blood pressure, and pulse measurements.

The WHO definition of biomarker includes "almost any measurement reflecting an interaction between a biological system and a potential hazard, which may be chemical, physical or biological. The measured response may be functional and physiological, biochemical at the cellular level, or a molecular interaction."

Clinical Endpoints have traditionally been the endpoints of all medical research. They reflect the patient's health from the patient's standpoint. Patients care about how they are doing, and how they feel, not the results of an individual blood test. The old expression, "The patient died, but the lab looked good," comes into mind. Patients want treatment for their diseases and conditions, not for an abnormal laboratory result. However, the alleviation of pain or an improvement in patient symptoms may not correlate with an improvement in the clinical course.

Biomarkers may serve as interim indicators before a clinical endpoint. The appropriate biomarker should be indicative of the fundamental clinical pathway. A clinical endpoint, such as survival, may take many years to determine, whereas the biomarker may provide interim evidence about the safety and efficacy of the treatment while the definitive data are being collected. The biomarker, as a surrogate endpoint, may identify dangerous or harmful treatments before the clinical endpoint is reached. They can result in more focused, and more efficient studies, at reduced expense. The most common biomarkers utilized in Alzheimer's disease and other types of dementia are bodily fluids and neuroimaging scans. What is needed are earlier, noninvasive, and inexpensive biomarkers.

Ocular Biomarkers

The optic nerve is considered the second cranial nerve of the peripheral nervous system but technically it is part of the central nervous system and not the peripheral nervous system. The myelin covering the nerves is produced by oligodendrocytes, not the Schwann cells of the peripheral nervous system. It is formed during the seventh week of embryonic development by the diencephalon. Peripheral nerves are sheathed by epineurium, perineurium, and endoneurium, and the optic nerve is covered by meningeal layers, dura, arachnoid, and pia mater.

For this reason, the eye may be an early biomarker for Alzheimer's disease.

Retinal thinning and optic nerve atrophy have been reported in patients with Alzheimer's disease. Aβ deposition has also been observed in the lens and retina. Amyloid plaques in the retina correlate with those found in the brain. Abnormalities in tear flow rate and function have also been reported. Thus, there are multiple avenues for research in the use of the eye as a biomarker for Alzheimer's disease.

Further Reading

Armstrong RA, Syed AB. Alzheimer's disease and the eye. Ophthalmic Physiol Opt. 2008;16:S2–8. https://doi.org/10.1111/j.1475-1313.1996.95001344.x.

Ashok A, Singh N, Chaudhary S, Bellamkonda V, Kritikos AE, Wise AS, Rana N, McDonald D, Ayyagari R. Retinal degeneration and Alzheimer's disease: an evolving link. Int J Mol Sci. 2020;21(19):7290. https://doi.org/10.3390/ijms21197290. PMID: 33023198; PMCID: PMC7582766.

Cheung CY, Mok V, Foster PJ, Trucco E, Chen C, Wong TY. Retinal imaging in Alzheimer's disease. J Neurol Neurosurg Psychiatry. 2021;92(9):983–94. https://doi.org/10.1136/jnnp-2020-325347. Epub 2021 Jun 9. PMID: 34108266.

Choi SI, Lee B, Woo JH, Jeong JB, Jun I, Kim EK. APP processing and metabolism in corneal fibroblasts and epithelium as a potential biomarker for Alzheimer's disease. Exp Eye Res. 2019;182:167–74. https://doi.org/10.1016/j.exer.2019.03.012.

Crooke A, Huete-Toral F, Martı A, Colligris B, Pintor J. Ocular disorders and the utility of animal models in the discovery of melatoninergic drugs with therapeutic potential. Expert Opin Drug Discov. 2012;7:989–1001. https://doi.org/10.1517/17460441.2012.714769.

Dutescu RM, Li QX, Crowston J, Masters CL, Baird PN, Culvenor JG. Amyloid precursor protein processing and retinal pathology in mouse models of Alzheimer's disease. Graefes Arch Clin Exp Ophthalmol. 2009;247:1213–21. https://doi.org/10.1007/s00417-009-1060-3.

Goldstein LE, Muffat JA, Cherny RA, Moir RD, Ericsson MH, Huang X, Mavros C, Coccia JA, Faget KY, Fitch KA, et al. Cytosolic β-amyloid deposition and supranuclear cataracts in lenses from people with Alzheimer's disease. Lancet. 2003;361:1258–65. https://doi.org/10.1016/S0140-6736(03)12981-9.

Kalló G, Emri M, Varga Z, Ujhelyi B, Tozsér J, Csutak A, Csosz É. Changes in the chemical barrier composition of tears in Alzheimer's disease reveal potential tear diagnostic biomarkers. PLoS One. 2016;11:1–14. https://doi.org/10.1371/journal.pone.0158000.

Kerbage C, Sadowsky CH, Tariot PN, Agronin M, Alva G, Turner FD, Nilan D, Cameron A, Cagle GD, Hartung PD. Detection of amyloid β signature in the lens and its correlation in the brain to aid in the diagnosis of Alzheimer's disease. Am J Alzheimers Dis Other Dement. 2015;30:738–45. https://doi.org/10.1177/1533317513520214.

Klyucherev TO, Olszewski P, Shalimova AA, Chubarev VN, Tarasov VV, Attwood MM, Syvänen S, Schiöth HB. Advances in the development of new biomarkers for Alzheimer's disease. Transl Neurodegener. 2022;11(1):25. https://doi.org/10.1186/s40035-022-00296-z. PMID: 35449079; PMCID: PMC9027827.

Koronyo Y, Rentsendorj A, Mirzaei N, Regis GC, Sheyn J, Shi H, Barron E, Cook-Wiens G, Rodriguez AR, Medeiros R, Paulo JA, Gupta VB, Kramerov AA, Ljubimov AV, Van Eyk JE, Graham SL, Gupta VK, Ringman JM, Hinton DR, Miller CA, Black KL, Cattaneo A, Meli G, Mirzaei M, Fuchs DT, Koronyo-Hamaoui M. Retinal pathological features and proteome signatures of Alzheimer's disease. Acta Neuropathol. 2023;145(4):409–38. https://doi.org/10.1007/s00401-023-02548-2. Epub 2023 Feb 11. PMID: 36773106; PMCID: PMC10020290.

Koronyo-Hamaoui M, Koronyo Y, Ljubimov AV, Miller CA, Ko MK, Black KL, Schwartz M, Farkas DL. Identification of amyloid plaques in retinas from Alzheimer's patients and noninvasive in vivo optical imaging of retinal plaques in a mouse model. NeuroImage. 2011;54:S204–17. https://doi.org/10.1016/j.neuroimage.2010.06.020.

More SS, Vince R. Hyperspectral imaging signatures detect amyloidopathy in Alzheimers mouse retina well before onset of cognitive decline. ACS Chem Neurosci. 2015;6:306–15. https://doi.org/10.1021/cn500242z.

Ning A, Cui J, To E, Ashe KH, Matsubara J. Amyloid-β deposits lead to retinal degeneration in a mouse model of Alzheimer disease. Investig Ophthalmol Vis Sci. 2008;49:5136–43. https://doi.org/10.1167/iovs.08-1849.

Örnek N, Dag E, Örnek K. Corneal sensitivity and tear function in neurodegenerative diseases. Curr Eye Res. 2015;40:423–8. https://doi.org/10.3109/02713683.2014.930154.

Romaus-Sanjurjo D, Regueiro U, López-López M, Vázquez-Vázquez L, Ouro A, Lema I, Sobrino T. Alzheimer's disease seen through the eye: ocular alterations and neurodegeneration. Int J Mol Sci. 2022;23(5):2486. https://doi.org/10.3390/ijms23052486. PMID: 35269629; PMCID: PMC8910735.

Singh AK, Verma S. Use of ocular biomarkers as a potential tool for early diagnosis of Alzheimer's disease. Indian J Ophthalmol. 2020;68:555–61.

Snyder PJ, Alber J, Alt C, Bain LJ, Bouma BE, Bouwman FH, DeBuc DC, Campbell MCW, Carrillo MC, Chew EY, Cordeiro MF, Dueñas MR, Fernández BM, Koronyo-Hamaoui M, La Morgia C, Carare RO, Sadda SR, van Wijngaarden P, Snyder HM. Retinal imaging in Alzheimer's and neurodegenerative diseases. Alzheimers Dement. 2021;17(1):103–11. https://doi.org/10.1002/alz.12179. Epub 2020 Oct 8. PMID: 33090722; PMCID: PMC8062064.

van Wijngaarden P, Hadoux X, Alwan M, Keel S, Dirani M. Emerging ocular biomarkers of Alzheimer disease. Clin Exp Ophthalmol. 2017;45:54–61. https://doi.org/10.1111/ceo.12872.

Zhang J, Shi L, Shen Y. The retina: a window in which to view the pathogenesis of Alzheimer's disease. Ageing Res Rev. 2022;77:101590. https://doi.org/10.1016/j.arr.2022.101590. Epub 2022 Feb 19. PMID: 35192959.

Chapter 2
Diagnosis

Biochemical/Neuroimaging

Recruiting

Sweden

The Swedish BioFINDER 2 Study (BioFINDER2)

ClinicalTrials.gov ID NCT03174938

Sponsor Skane University Hospital
Information provided by Oskar Hansson, Skane University Hospital (Responsible Party)
Last Update Posted 2021-03-02

Brief Summary

The Swedish BioFINDER 2 study is a new study that was launched in 2017 and extended the previous cohorts of BioFINDER 1 study (www.biofinder.se). BioFINDER 1 is used, e.g., to characterize the role of beta-amyloid pathology in early diagnosis of Alzheimer's disease (AD) using amyloid-PET (18F-Flutemetamol) and Aβ analysis in cerebrospinal fluid samples. The BioFINDER 1 study has resulted in more than 40 publications during the last 3 years, many in high-impact journals, and some of the results have already had important implications for the diagnostic work-up of patients with AD in the clinical routine practice.

The original BioFINDER 1 cohort started to include participants in 2008. Since then, there has been a rapid development of biochemical and neuroimaging technologies that enable novel ways to study biological processes involved in Alzheimer's disease in living people. There has also been a growing interest in the earliest stages of AD and other neurodegenerative diseases. With the advent of new tau-PET tracers, there is now an opportunity to elucidate the role of tau pathology in the

J. N. Weiss, *Alzheimer's Disease and the Eye*,
https://doi.org/10.1007/978-3-031-58811-2_2

pathogenesis of AD and other tauopathies. The Swedish BioFINDER 2 study has been designed to complement the BioFINDER 1 study and to, e.g., address issues regarding the role of tau pathology in different dementias and in preclinical stages of different dementia diseases. Further, the clinical assessments and MRI methods have been further optimized compared to BioFINDER 1.

Detailed Description

General Aims

1. Develop methods for early and accurate diagnosis of different dementia disorders. This is important not only for the clinical diagnostic work-up, but also for the selection of patients to clinical trials. Because dementia is very common among the elderly, but often misdiagnosed, we need to develop minimally invasive, reliable, and affordable biomarkers for use in a primary care setting. This could include blood-based biomarkers which could be used to identify patients at high risk for a neurodegenerative disease. We also aim to develop new diagnostic algorithms using advanced imaging techniques and cerebrospinal fluid (CSF) biomarkers to diagnose patients prior to overt symptoms (when brain dysfunction is still limited and potentially reversible) in order to identify individuals more likely to respond to new disease-modifying therapies.

2. Develop biomarkers and imaging techniques to monitor the early effects of new disease-modifying therapies. Methods are needed that can reliably detect relevant changes in the turnover of Aβ, tau, and α-synuclein. In the present study, one focus will be to study the annual change in the retention of Tau PET ligands during both the prodromal and dementia stages of AD. Further, we need biomarkers that detect the intensity of ongoing synaptic/neuronal degeneration. Imaging methods revealing the functional and structural integrity of different brain networks might also be relevant.

3. Investigate the heterogeneity of dementia and Parkinsonian disorders to assist in the development of a new pathology-based disease classification. The current diagnostic work-up is based on symptomatology. However, the diseases (e.g., Alzheimer's and Parkinson's diseases) are heterogeneous with respect to clinical features and underlying pathologies. Moreover, there is also significant overlap between the diseases. Hence, today's symptom-based clinical diagnostic criteria are likely too crude to provide an etiologically meaningful classification of patients. We will therefore work toward a pathology-based disease classification, using in vivo biomarkers that reflect the underlying brain pathologies, e.g., Aβ or tau. This will be especially useful for the development of new disease-modifying therapies, which are aimed at specific brain pathologies.

4. Define the temporal evolution of pathologies in the predementia phases of Alzheimer's disease. One of the last decade's paradigm shifts in neuroscience has been the realization that AD, and likely also other neurodegenerative diseases, starts with a prolonged predementia phase. AD even starts with an asymptomatic phase, when brain pathology is present in the absence of clinical symptoms. It has become clear that we need to better understand the temporal

sequence of pathologic events in these disorders to be able to select the optimal disease stages for interventions in clinical trials with different disease-modifying therapies directed at specific pathologies.

5. Investigate the underlying disease mechanisms of dementia disorders in humans aiming at finding new relevant drug targets. Drug discovery using the currently available cell and animal models has not translated to human research as indicated by failed phase II and III trials. There are several possible reasons for these failures. First, it is possible that previous trials may have focused on the wrong drug targets, since findings from cell and animal models of dementias may not have accurately captured essential aspects of the disease mechanisms in humans. BioFINDER2 will be a translational study where we will attempt to bridge the knowledge gap between cell/animal studies and studies in humans, by using biomarkers that reflect biological mechanisms that may be studied across model systems. Second, another reason for the failed trials may be that they included patients in too advanced disease stages for the treatments to be effective, or that they partly included patients with unspecific diseases, since they did not use biomarker-based methods for the inclusion of participants. BioFINDER2 will inform the design of future clinical trials by providing detailed data about cognitive and functional changes over time in people with well-defined biomarker-characterized brain pathologies.

Study Plan

To reach the objectives above, we include well-characterized and clinically relevant populations of patients with dementia and/or Parkinsonian symptoms and healthy individuals. We apply several state-of-the art methodologies in order to develop new brain imaging techniques, new biomarkers in blood and CSF as well as novel methods of assessing important clinical symptoms.

Cognitive Testing

Attention and executive function will be assessed with the Trail Making Test A and B (TMT), Symbol Digit Modalities Test (SDMT), and A Quick Test of cognitive speed (AQT). Visuospatial ability will be measured by two subtests from the Visual Objects and Space Perception (VOSP) battery, incomplete letters, and cube analysis. Memory will be assessed with the Free and Cued Selective Reminding Test (FCSRT) in cohorts A and B. It will be complemented with the ten-word delayed recall test from ADAS-cog, including a recognition part. Verbal ability will be evaluated with the animal and letter S fluency tests and the 15-item short version of the Boston Naming Test. Global cognition will be assessed with the Mini-Mental State Examination (MMSE). In cohorts A and B, a computerized cognitive battery focusing on memory and attention will also be performed.

Assessments of Symptoms, Functional Abilities, and Global Function

Cognitive symptoms. All subjects will rate his or her memory and attention/executive function in relation to others of the same age according to the Brief Anosognosia Scale (BAS). We have also added similar questions to cover the other cognitive domains. These questions have been validated against neuropsychological testing but data are indicating that self-reported cognitive complaints are only valid in a lesser degree of cognitive impairment. To assess a broader range of cognitive complaints, the Subjective Cognitive Decline questionnaire (SCD-q) will be administered to the research subjects. Subjects from cohorts C, D, and E will be assessed with a cognitive impairment questionnaire (CIMP-QUEST; filled out by an informant).

Functional ability. This will be evaluated with the informant-based Functional Activities Questionnaire (FAQ) or the Amsterdam IADL scale, both focusing on instrumental activities of daily living (IADL) known to be affected early in cognitive decline.

Global function. The global cognitive status will be evaluated using the sum of boxes score from the Clinical Dementia Rating Scale (CDR) and the Global Deterioration Scale (GDS).

Behavioral and psychological symptoms in dementia (BPSD). BPSD will be assessed by clinicians using the Neuropsychiatric Inventory—Clinician Rating Scale (NPI-C) developed by Jeffrey Cummings. Mood and anxiety will be further assessed with the Hospital Anxiety and Depression Scale (HADS). Frontal Behavioral Inventory (FBI) will be done in FTD-related conditions.

Quality of Life (QoL). The overall health status will be rated by the subjects using the EQ-5D from Euro-QoL. In demented patients, this will also be rated by an informant, spouse, or close relative.

Sleep. The presence of REM sleep behavior disorder will be evaluated with a single validated composite question derived from the Mayo Sleep Questionnaire. Sleep quality is assessed with the Sleep Scale from the Medical Outcome Study (MOS).

Cognitive reserve. Premorbid cognition and cognitive reserve are approximated from the Cognitive Reserve Index questionnaire (CRI-q; subitems "Education" and "Working activity," not "Leisure time").

Cerebrospinal Fluid (CSF), Blood Sampling, and Analysis
Lumbar CSF samples will be collected according to a standardized protocol and will follow the principles of the Alzheimer's Association Flow Chart for CSF biomarkers. In short, lumbar puncture will be done between 9 and 12 am. Twenty to thirty milliliters of CSF will be collected in low-binding polypropylene tubes, which are stored on ice for 5–20 min until the CSF samples are centrifuged ($2000 \times g$, $+4\ ^\circ\mathrm{C}$, 10 min). Thereafter, the CSF will be aliquoted in ca. 1 mL portions into low-binding polypropylene tubes followed by storage at $-80\ ^\circ\mathrm{C}$ until batch analyses.

Plasma collection will be done at the same visit as the lumbar puncture. Blood will be drawn into tubes containing either EDTA (5×6 mL tubes) or lithium heparin (3×3 mL tubes) as an anticoagulant. After centrifugation ($2000 \times g$, $+4\ ^\circ\mathrm{C}$, 10 min), plasma samples will be aliquoted into polypropylene tubes and stored at $-80\ ^\circ\mathrm{C}$ pending biochemical analyses. Further, EDTA-blood (2×6 mL) will also be obtained for genetic DNA analyses.

Magnetic Resonance Imaging

Three Tesla MRI (Siemens Prisma) will be done in all study cohorts. A wide variety of magnetic resonance imaging (MRI) techniques will be used to study regional brain volume (three-dimensional magnetization-prepared rapid acquisition with gradient echo (3D MPRAGE)), metabolism (MR spectroscopy (MRS)), structural and functional connectivity of different brain regions (diffusion tensor imaging (DTI) and functional MRI (fMRI)), regional blood flow (arterial spin labeling (ASL)), iron deposition (susceptibility-weighted imaging (SWI)), and the presence of small vessel disease (MPRAGE, SWI, and fluid-attenuated inversion recovery (FLAIR)). The protocol will take approximately 60 min to perform. No contrast-enhancing agent will be used.

PET Imaging

Tau PET. PET imaging of tau aggregates will be done in all the included cohorts at baseline. In the present study, Tau PET imaging will be performed using 18F-RO6958948 developed by Hoffmann-La Roche which will provide the precursor for this PET ligand. This tau PET imaging agent has been shown to accurately detect tau pathology in cases with AD when compared to controls. We will perform a 20–30 min PET scan approximately 60 min post intravenous injection of 18F-RO6958948. The impact of the investigation on clinical diagnostic accuracy and patient care will be investigated. 18F-RO6958948 has not yet been approved for use in clinical routine practice in Sweden, and can only be used in research studies, such as the present study.

Amyloid PET. PET imaging of Aβ aggregates (including 18F-flutemetamol PET) has been approved for use in clinical routine practice in Sweden. In the present study, 18F-flutemetamol PET will be done in nondemented cases only. In the cases with dementia, CSF Aβ will be enough to determine the presence or absence of brain amyloid pathology. However, in the cognitively healthy cases and in the patients with SCD or MCI, we are interested in following the spread of amyloid pathology throughout the brain during the preclinical stages of AD and the spatial relationship to tau pathology. Therefore, Amyloid PET will be done according to clinical routine procedures in addition to CSF Aβ measurements in these groups. In the present study, Amyloid PET will be performed using 18F-flutemetamol. GE Healthcare will provide the precursor for 18F-flutemetamol. A 20 min scan will be performed between 90 and 110 min post injection of 18F-flutemetamol.

FDOPA PET FDOPA

PET is often used as part of clinical routine examinations of patients with Parkinsonism to confirm the diagnosis. Here, DaTSCAN will be done according to clinical routine procedures in cases with PD, PDD, DLB, MSA, PSP, and CBD to confirm the clinical diagnosis if it has not been done in clinical routine praxis within 1 year from the baseline visit.

Official Title
The Swedish BioFINDER 2 Study

Conditions
Dementia
Alzheimer Disease
Parkinson Disease
Lewy Body Disease
Parkinson-Dementia Syndrome
Frontotemporal Degeneration
Semantic Dementia
Progressive Nonfluent Aphasia
Progressive Supranuclear Palsy
Corticobasal Degeneration
Multiple System Atrophy
Mild Cognitive Impairment
Show fewer conditions

Intervention/Treatment
- Diagnostic Test: Flutemetamol F18 Injection
- Diagnostic Test: [18F]-RO6958948
- Diagnostic Test: Elecsys (Roche) Abeta42, Ttau and Ptau
- Diagnostic Test: Lumipulse (Fujirebio) Abeta42, Ttau and Ptau

Other Study ID Numbers
- BioFINDER 2

Study Start (Actual)
2017-05-15

Primary Completion (Estimated)
2028-12-31

Study Completion (Estimated)
2028-12-31

Enrollment (Estimated)
1505

Study Type
Interventional

Phase
Not Applicable

Study Contact
Name: Oskar Hansson, MD, Professor
Phone Number: +46 (0)40335036
Email: oskar.hansson@med.lu.se

Study Contact Backup
Name: Erik Stomrud, MD, PhD
Email: erik.stomrud@med.lu.se
Sweden

Malmö, Sweden, SE-20502
Recruiting
Memory Clinic, Skåne University Hospital

Contact
Erik Stomrud, MD, PhD
erik.stomrud@med.lu.se

Ängelholm, Sweden, SE-262 81
Not yet recruiting
Memory Clinic, Hospital of Ängelholm

Contact
Per Johansson, MD, PhD

Contact
per.a.johansson@skane.se

Eligibility Criteria

Description

Cohort A: Cognitively healthy younger individuals (40–65 years of age)

Inclusion Criteria
- Age 40–65 years
- Absence of cognitive symptoms as assessed by a physician with special interest in cognitive disorders
- MMSE score 27–30 at screening visit
- Do not fulfill the criteria for MCI or any dementia according to DSM-V
- Speaks and understands Swedish to the extent that an interpreter is not necessary for the patient to fully understand the study information and cognitive tests

Exclusion Criteria
- Significant unstable systemic illness or organ failure, such as terminal cancer, that makes it difficult to participate in the study
- Current significant alcohol or substance misuse
- Significant neurological or psychiatric illness
- Refusing lumbar puncture, MRI, or PET

Cohort B: Cognitively healthy elderly individuals (66–100 years of age).

Inclusion Criteria
- Age 66–100 years
- Absence of cognitive symptoms as assessed by a physician with a special interest in cognitive disorders

- MMSE score 26–30 at screening visit
- Do not fulfill the criteria for MCI or any dementia according to DSM-V
- Speaks and understands Swedish to the extent that an interpreter is not necessary for the patient to fully understand the study information and cognitive tests

Exclusion Criteria
- Significant unstable systemic illness or organ failure, such as terminal cancer, that makes it difficult to participate in the study.
- Current significant alcohol or substance misuse.
- Significant neurological or psychiatric illness.
- Refusing lumbar puncture, MRI, or PET.

Cohort C: Subjective cognitive decline and mild cognitive impairment.

Inclusion Criteria
- Age 40–100 years.
- Referred to the memory clinics due to cognitive symptoms experienced by the patient and/or informant. These symptoms do not have to be memory complaints, but could also be executive, visuospatial, language, praxis, psychomotor, or social-cognitive complaints.
- MMSE score of 24–30 points.
- Do not fulfill the criteria for any dementia (major neurocognitive disorder) according to DSM-V.
- The medical doctor (after clinical assessments, cognitive testing, CSF analyses, and structural brain imaging) believes the cognitive complaints are caused by an incipient neurocognitive disorder of any sort. This is defined as any case fulfilling the criteria above (i.e., both SCD and MCI) with an abnormal CSF Aβ42/40 ratio, which is strongly associated with brain Aβ pathology and prodromal Alzheimer's disease. Furthermore, cases with MCI (=minor neurocognitive impairment) due to either Parkinson's disease, Lewy body disease, vascular neurocognitive disorder, or frontotemporal dementia can also be included.
- Speaks and understands Swedish to the extent that an interpreter is not necessary for the patient to fully understand the study information and cognitive tests.

Exclusion Criteria
- Significant unstable systemic illness or organ failure, such as terminal cancer, that makes it difficult to participate in the study.
- Current significant alcohol or substance misuse.
- Refusing lumbar puncture, MRI, or PET.

Cohort D: Dementia due to Alzheimer's disease.

Inclusion Criteria
- Age 40–100 years.
- Referred to the memory clinics due to cognitive symptoms experienced by the patient and/or informant. These symptoms do not have to be memory complaints,

but could also be executive, visuospatial, language, praxis, or psychomotor complaints.

- MMSE score of 12–26 points.
- Fulfill the criteria for dementia (major neurocognitive disorder) due to Alzheimer's disease (DSM-V).
- Speaks and understands Swedish to the extent that an interpreter was not necessary for the patient to fully understand the study information and cognitive tests.

Exclusion Criteria

- Significant unstable systemic illness or organ failure, such as terminal cancer, that makes it difficult to participate in the study.
- Current significant alcohol or substance misuse.
- Refusing lumbar puncture, MRI, or PET.

Cohort E: Other dementias.

Inclusion Criteria

- Age 40–100 years.
- Fulfill the criteria for dementia (major neurocognitive disorder) due to FTD, PDD, DLB, or subcortical VaD alternatively the criteria for PD, PSP, MSA, or CBS.
- Speaks and understands Swedish to the extent that an interpreter was not necessary for the patient to fully understand the study information and cognitive tests.

Exclusion Criteria

- Significant unstable systemic illness or organ failure, such as terminal cancer, that makes it difficult to participate in the study.
- Current significant alcohol or substance misuse.
- Refusing lumbar puncture, MRI, or PET.

Ages Eligible for Study

20 Years to 100 Years (Adult, Older Adult)

Sexes Eligible for Study

All

Accepts Healthy Volunteers

Yes

Design Details

Primary Purpose: Diagnostic
Allocation: Non-Randomized
Interventional Model: Single Group Assignment
Masking: None (Open Label)

Arms and interventions

Participant group/arm	Intervention/treatment
Other: Cohort A: Cognitively healthy younger individuals (40–65 years) We will recruit 300 cognitively healthy individuals from the Malmö Offspring study, which is an epidemiological study. The participants will be stratified according to (a) family history of dementia in first degree relatives (with onset before 80 years of age) and (b) APOE 4 genotype; i.e., 25% will have no family history and no APOE4 allele, 25% will have a family history and no APOE 4 allele, 25% will have no family history and at least one APOE 4 allele, 25% will have a family history and at least one APOE 4 allele FOLLOW-UP FOR 8 YEARS Every 2 years new clinical, cognitive, neurological, and psychiatric assessments will be performed as well as CSF/blood sampling MRI, Tau PET and Amyloid PET will be done every 4 years in all cases, and Tau PET and MRI every 2 years if the subject is amyloid positive at baseline. An auxiliary cohort (termed "Cohort A2") of 40 healthy individuals aged 20–40 years of age will also be included	Diagnostic Test: Flutemetamol F18 Injection • PET imaging of Abeta amyloid • Other names: – Vizamyl Diagnostic Test: [18F]-RO6958948 • PET imaging of Tau aggregates Diagnostic Test: Elecsys (Roche) Abeta42, Ttau and Ptau • Measurement of Abeta42, Ttau, and Ptau in the cerebrospinal fluid Diagnostic Test: Lumipulse (Fujirebio) Abeta42, Ttau, and Ptau • Measurement of Abeta42, Ttau, and Ptau in the cerebrospinal fluid
Other: Cohort B: Cognitively healthy elderly individuals (66–100 years) We will recruit 300 cognitively healthy individuals from the Malmö/Lund region, where we will aim to include as many individuals as possible who participated in the Malmö Diet and Cancer study during the early 1990s. The participants will be stratified according to (a) family history of dementia in first degree relatives (with onset before 80 years of age) and (b) APOE 4 genotype; i.e., 25% will have no family history and no APOE 4 allele, 25% will have a family history and no APOE 4 allele, 25% will have no family history and at least one APOE 4 allele, 25% will have a family history and at least one APOE 4 allele FOLLOW-UP FOR 8 YEARS Every 2 years new clinical, cognitive, neurological, and psychiatric assessments will be performed as well as CSF/blood sampling MRI, Tau PET and Amyloid PET will be done every 4 years in all cases, and Tau PET and MRI every 2 years if the subject is amyloid positive at baseline	Diagnostic Test: Flutemetamol F18 Injection • PET imaging of Abeta amyloid • Other names: – Vizamyl Diagnostic Test: [18F]-RO6958948 • PET imaging of Tau aggregates Diagnostic Test: Elecsys (Roche) Abeta42, Ttau, and Ptau • Measurement of Abeta42, Ttau, and Ptau in the cerebrospinal fluid Diagnostic Test: Lumipulse (Fujirebio) Abeta42, Ttau, and Ptau • Measurement of Abeta42, Ttau, and Ptau in the cerebrospinal fluid

Participant group/arm	Intervention/treatment
Other: Cohort C: SCD and MCI Five hundred and fifty patients with either subjective cognitive decline or mild cognitive impairment will be recruited in a consecutive fashion from the Skåne University Hospital and Ängelholm Hospital. We will only include cases where the medical doctor believes that the cognitive symptoms are caused by an incipient neurocognitive disorder. For example, all cases with evidence of brain amyloid pathology (i.e., an abnormal CSF Aβ42/40 ratio) will be included FOLLOW-UP FOR 6 YEARS Every 12 months new clinical, cognitive, neurological, and psychiatric assessments will be performed CSF/blood sampling, Tau PET (depends on further funding) and MRI will be done every 2 years. Amyloid PET will be performed at baseline and after 4 years An auxiliary cohort ("Cohort C2") 150 cases with SCD/MCI where the doctor does not suspect incipient neurocognitive disorder, will undergo the same baseline investigations, but they will be followed up clinically only after 2, 4 and 8 years	Diagnostic Test: Flutemetamol F18 Injection • PET imaging of Abeta amyloid • Other names: – Vizamyl Diagnostic Test: [18F]-RO6958948 • PET imaging of Tau aggregates Diagnostic Test: Elecsys (Roche) Abeta42, Ttau, and Ptau • Measurement of Abeta42, Ttau, and Ptau in the cerebrospinal fluid Diagnostic Test: Lumipulse (Fujirebio) Abeta42, Ttau and Ptau • Measurement of Abeta42, Ttau, and Ptau in the cerebrospinal fluid
Other: Cohort D: Dementia due to Alzheimer's disease Three hundred patients with mild to moderate dementia due to Alzheimer's disease (AD) will be recruited from the Skåne University Hospital and Ängelholm Hospital in southern Sweden. We will include 50 cases aged 40–65 years of age, 200 cases aged 66–79 years of age, and 50 cases aged 80–100 years of age FOLLOW-UP FOR 2 YEARS Every 12 months new clinical, cognitive, neurological, and psychiatric assessments will be performed CSF/blood sampling, Tau PET (depends on further funding) and MRI will be done at baseline and after 2 years. No Amyloid PET in this group	Diagnostic Test: [18F]-RO6958948 • PET imaging of Tau aggregates Diagnostic Test: Elecsys (Roche) Abeta42, Ttau and Ptau • Measurement of Abeta42, Ttau, and Ptau in the cerebrospinal fluid Diagnostic Test: Lumipulse (Fujirebio) Abeta42, Ttau, and Ptau • Measurement of Abeta42, Ttau, and Ptau in the cerebrospinal fluid

Participant group/arm	Intervention/treatment

Other: Cohort E: Other dementias
Patients with primary neurodegenerative disorders other than Alzheimer's disease will be recruited:
  1. 160 cases with frontotemporal dementia (FTD)-related disorders, including behavioral variant of FTD (bvFTD), progressive nonfluent aphasia (PNFA), semantic dementia (SD), progressive supranuclear palsy (PSP), corticobasal degeneration (CBD)
  2. 50 cases with subcortical vascular dementia (VaD)
  3. 200 cases with either Parkinson's disease (PD), Parkinson's disease with dementia (PDD), dementia with Lewy Bodies (DLB), Multiple system atrophy (MSA)
FOLLOW-UP FOR 2 YEARS Every 12 months new clinical, cognitive, neurological, and psychiatric assessments will be performed CSF/blood sampling, Tau PET (depends on further funding) and MRI will be done at baseline and after 2 years. No Amyloid PET in this group
	Diagnostic Test: [18F]-RO6958948
	  • PET imaging of Tau aggregates
	Diagnostic Test: Elecsys (Roche) Abeta42, Ttau, and Ptau
	  • Measurement of Abeta42, Ttau, and Ptau in the cerebrospinal fluid
	Diagnostic Test: Lumipulse (Fujirebio) Abeta42, Ttau, and Ptau
	  • Measurement of Abeta42, Ttau, and Ptau in the cerebrospinal fluid

Primary outcome measures

Outcome measure	Measure description	Time frame
Clinical diagnosis	Clinical diagnosis according to consensus group decision blinded to the diagnostic test	Clinical diagnosis at last 1 day visit
Clinical Dementia Rating-Sum of Boxes (CDR-SB)	Change in CDR-SB	Time zero equals the baseline visit. All subjects will subsequently attend follow-up visits every year for approximately 2–8 years after baseline

Secondary outcome measures

Outcome measure	Measure description	Time frame
Rate of cognitive decline as measured by MMSE	Mini Mental State Examination (MMSE)	Time zero equals the baseline visit. All subjects will subsequently attend follow-up visits every year for approximately 2–8 years after baseline
Rate of cognitive decline as measured in ADL function	ADL function will be determined using the Functional Assessment Questionnaire (FAQ) and The Amsterdam ADL scale	Time zero equals the baseline visit. All subjects will subsequently attend follow-up visits every year for approximately 2–8 years after baseline

Outcome measure	Measure description	Time frame
Rate of volume change of structural MRI measures and amyloid PET		Time zero equals the baseline visit. All subjects will subsequently attend follow-up visits every year for approximately 2–8 years after baseline
Rates of change on cerebrospinal fluid AD biomarkers		Time zero equals the baseline visit. All subjects will subsequently attend follow-up visits every year for approximately 2–8 years after baseline

Sponsor

Skane University Hospital

Collaborators

- Lund University

Investigators

- Principal Investigator: Oskar Hansson, MD, Professor, Skåne University Hospital, and Lund University

General Publications

No publications available

Cognitive Decline

Recruiting

Italy

PRedicting the EVolution of SubjectIvE Cognitive Decline to Alzheimer's Disease with Machine Learning (PREVIEW)

ClinicalTrials.gov ID NCT05569083

Sponsor Azienda Ospedaliero-Universitaria Careggi
Information provided by Valentina Bessi, Azienda Ospedaliero-Universitaria Careggi (Responsible Party)
Last Update Posted 2022-10-07

Brief Summary

Alzheimer's disease (AD) has a presymptomatic course which can last from several years to decades. Identification of subjects at an early stage is crucial for therapeutic intervention and possible prevention of cognitive decline. Current research is focused on identifying characteristics of the early stages of AD and several concepts have been developed to that end.

Subjective cognitive decline (SCD) is defined as a self-experienced persistent decline in cognitive capacity in comparison with the subject's previously normal status, during which the subject has normal age-, gender-, and education-adjusted performance on standardized cognitive tests. SCD is not related to current cognitive impairment, however, it has been considered for its potential role as risk factors for AD.

The aim of this study is to evaluate, through machine learning tools, the accuracy data, neuropsychological assessment, personality traits, cognitive reserve, genetic factors, cerebrospinal fluid (CSF) neurodegeneration biomarkers, EEG, and Event Related Potential recordings in predicting conversion from SCD condition, to Mild Cognitive Impairment (MCI) and AD.

Detailed Description

The Regional Reference Center for Alzheimer's Disease and Cognitive Disorders of Careggi Hospital, Florence, started about 25 years ago to collect clinical, neuropsychological, personality, and lifestyle data for patients with of Subjective Cognitive Decline (SCD). Starting from these data, the aim of the present study is to increase the number of variables collected on SCD subjects and expand the clinical follow-up to delineate a more accurate pathway of disease and to identify very early subjects at risk of conversion in Alzheimer's Disease (AD).

The advantages of detection of cognitive impairment at the early stages are critical. Such detection has traditionally been performed manually by one or more clinicians based on reports and test results. Machine learning algorithms offer a method of detection that may provide an automated process and valuable insights into diagnosis and classification. With this tool clinicians could design optimal screenings to predict, already at the stage of SCD, possible evolutions of the patient's conditions, and, through decisional protocols, establish the degree of appropriateness of the investigations/exam to perform for each patient, based on the current state of risk.

The aim of this study is to evaluate, through machine learning tools, the accuracy of clinical data, neuropsychological assessment, personality traits, cognitive reserve, genetic factors, cerebrospinal fluid (CSF) neurodegeneration biomarkers, and features from EEG and event-related potentials (ERP) in predicting conversion from SCD condition, to Mild Cognitive Impairment (MCI) and AD.

All participants will undergo a comprehensive familial and clinical history, general and neurological examination, extensive neuropsychological battery (about 19 tests exploring all cognitive domains: memory, attention, executive functions, language, praxis), estimation of premorbid intelligence (TIB—Test di Intelligenza Breve, an Italian version of the National Adult Reading Test—NART), personality traits (Big Five Factors Questionnaire—BFFQ), and leisure activities evaluation (structured interviewed regarding participation in intellectual, sporting, and social activities) as well as assessment of depression (Hamilton Depression Rating Scale—HDRS). Moreover, all patients will undergo a CSF analysis to assess established biomarkers (Aβ42, total tau, p-tau), and blood samples for DNA analysis will be collected to identify the Apolipoprotein E (APOE) and brain-derived neurotrophic factor (BDNF) genotypes. In particular, three different single nucleotide polymorphisms (SNPs) will be analyzed:

- BDNF SNP Val66Met (valine-methionine substitution) was already associated with poorer episodic memory and abnormal hippocampal activation assayed with MRI.
- APOE genes rs429358 and rs7412 are involved in the Amyloid plaque formation. Only clinical and neuropsychological assessments are repeated yearly in order to evaluate the progression of decline.

The sub-sample will be selected including all new cases of SCD included in the study (about 50), all subjects converted to MCI (about 25), and all patients, already studied, who report a subjective cognitive disorder for less than 10 years (about 75).

This selected sub-sample will also perform additional investigations: CSF biomarkers, resting state EEG recordings, and ERP registration.

For about 150 subjects, the EEG activity will be recorded. The participants will be administered an ERP test battery with concurrently recorded EEG. Analysis of EEG data, in particular, will start with a standardized early-stage EEG processing pipeline (PREP Pipeline) focusing on high-filtering at 1 Hz, the identification of bad channels, and the calculation of a robust average reference. The investigators will perform signal epoching using fixed-length epochs for resting state measurements and stimulus-locked epochs for signals acquired during tasks. Epochs containing artifactual signals will be removed with a semi-automatic procedure. The investigators will then apply independent component analysis (ICA) to the data, followed by a semiautomatic detection of artifactual components based on measures of autocorrelation, correlation with the EOG electrode, focal channel topography, and quality of mono-source dipole fitting. Finally, the investigators will compute power features at the sensor space, i.e. frequency bands powers, and linear/non-linear functional connectivity metrics, i.e., direct transfer function and mutual information, at the source level after a source reconstruction procedure, i.e., Low-Resolution Brain Electromagnetic Tomography (LORETA) method.

Machine learning analysis will proceed as follows. The first analysis will include all the patients who were diagnosed with SCD in the preliminary work. The investigators will define a set of multi-modal features including all the 19 neuropsychological tests, a selection of the personality assessments, and the genetic profile. The investigators will define common metrics based on the dispersion of every single dimension of the profile and then they will train a machine learning algorithm to associate each profile "vector" to the associated evolution of the disease after a fixed time (at first the possible categories will be only SCD, MCI, AD with no further sublevels, but this can be improved in further rounds). First, the investigators will perform this classification with standard machine learning procedures such as support vector machine (SVM, using binary decision trees) and k-nearest neighbors (kNN). Then they will exploit the fact that neurophysiological assessments are repeated yearly (see above) to use the SuStaIn algorithm previously applied to neuroimaging data (see state of the art). Briefly, the algorithm z-scores each dimension of the profile and models with a piece-wise linear function the different paths of accumulations of each marker, i.e., the progression from healthy to abnormal values. This approach does not only outperform standard algorithms in predicting the final condition of the subjects based on the starting profile but highlights the different paths that can lead to the same outcome. In a separate set of analyses, the investigators will follow a deep learning approach, using exactly the same subject profiles to train a multi-level feedforward artificial neural network (ANN) predicting the condition of the patient after a fixed time. The networks will be trained with standard gradient descent and backpropagation techniques, and by means of dropout and batch normalization procedures the investigators will obtain robust automatic classification results. Comparing SuStaIn and ANN classification performance they will decide the most convenient approach for the task. Moreover, they will apply standard dimensionality reduction techniques to extract the most salient features and repeat the procedure described above to assess whether it is possible to achieve the same results with a subset of the screenings.

The selected approach will be then repeated to the novel patients recruited during PREVIEW and those undergoing follow-up analysis during the project. The only difference will be the novel set of factors included in the analysis, including all the data used in the first version but also BDNF, CSF biomarkers, and the novel features extracted from resting state EEG recordings and ERP. This will require defining a second multi-modal metric across all features, and a consequent reshaping and retraining of the machine learning network. As described above, even for the second version of the algorithm the investigators will aim at defining the minimal set of features achieving the optimal performance. The final outcome of the algorithm will provide a prediction of the evolution of the condition for each patient based on his/her complete profile.

Official Title
PRedicting the EVolution of SubjectIvE Cognitive Decline to Alzheimer's Disease
   with Machine Learning

Conditions
Cognitive Decline
Mild Cognitive Impairment
Alzheimer Disease

Intervention/Treatment
- Genetic: Genetic analysis of APOE and BDNF genes
- Diagnostic Test: EEG recording
- Diagnostic Test: CSF collection and AD biomarker measurement

- Diagnostic Test: Neuropsychological evaluation
- Diagnostic Test: Assessment of cognitive reserve, depression, personality traits, and leisure activities
- Diagnostic Test: Clinical-neuropsychological follow-up
- Diagnostic Test: ERP recording

Other Study ID Numbers
- 20RSVB

Study Start (Actual)
2020-10-01

Primary Completion (Estimated)
2023-09-30

Study Completion (Estimated)
2024-03-30

Enrollment (Estimated)
350

Study Type
Observational

Study Contact
Name: Valentina Bessi, MD, PhD
Phone Number: +393496096308
Email: valentina.bessi@unifi.it

Study Contact Backup
Name: Sonia Padiglioni, Psy, PhD
Phone Number: +393488512232
Email: padiglionis@aou-careggi.toscana.it
Italy

Florence, Italy, 50143
Recruiting
IRCCS Don Gnocchi

Contact
Antonello Grippo, MD, PhD

Principal Investigator
Sandro Sorbi, MD, PhD

Florence, Italy
Recruiting
Department of Neuroscience, Psychology, Drug Research and Child Health,
    University of Florence

Contact
Benedetta Nacmias, PhD
055/7948910 nacmias@unifi.it

Principal Investigator
Benedetta Nacmias, PhD

Pisa, Italy
Recruiting
Istituto di Biorobotica e Dipartimento di Eccellenza in Robotica e AI, Scuola
    Superiore Sant'Anna

Contact
Alberto Mazzoni, PhD

Principal Investigator
Alberto Mazzoni

Tuscany Region Locations

Florence, Tuscany Region, Italy, 50134
Recruiting
AOU Careggi

Contact
Valentina Bessi, MD, PhD
+393496096308 valentina.bessi@unifi.it

Contact
Salvatore Mazzeo, MD
+393477219137 salvatore.mazzeo@unifi.it

Principal Investigator
Valentina Bessi, MD, PhD

Inclusion Criteria
- Complaining of cognitive decline with a duration of ≥ 6 months
- Normal functioning on the Activities of Daily Living and the Instrumental Activities of Daily Living scales
- Unsatisfied criteria for dementia at baseline (DSM-V)

Exclusion Criteria
- History of head injury, current neurological and/or systemic disease, symptoms of psychosis, major depression, alcoholism, or other substance abuse

Study Population
The investigators will include in the study, consecutive spontaneous subjects who self-referred to the Centre for Alzheimer's Disease and Adult Cognitive Disorders of Careggi Hospital in Florence.

The investigators will include in the study 300 patients with SCD already selected and evaluated one time (baseline) or more (follow-up) in our clinic, and they will increase the baseline sample by adding new subjects with SCD or MCI.

Ages Eligible for Study
- (Child, Adult, Older Adult)

Sexes Eligible for Study
- All

Accepts Healthy Volunteers
- Yes

Sampling Method
- Non-Probability Sample

Design Details
- Observational Model: Cohort
Time Perspective: Prospective
Biospecimen Retention: Samples with DNA
Biospecimen Description: CSF biomarkers, whole blood

Cohorts and interventions

Group/cohort	Intervention/treatment
Patients with Subjective Cognitive Decline Patients complaining about cognitive decline with normal functioning in the activities of daily living and unsatisfied criteria for MCI or dementia at baseline	Genetic: genetic analysis of APOE and BDNF genes • The three SNPs (rs429358, rs7412, and rs6265 on APOE and BDNF genes respectively) will be analyzed by the polymerase chain reaction (PCR) on genomic DNA and with the analysis of melting curves (HRMA) using the Rotor-Gene 6000 (Rotor-Gene, Corbett Research, Mortlake, Australia) Diagnostic test: EEG recording • The EEG activity will be recorded continuously from 19 sites by using electrodes set in an elastic cap and positioned according to the 10–20 international system. The recording will be referenced to the common average of all electrodes, excluding Fp1 and Fp2. Re-referencing will be done prior to the EEG artifact detection and analysis. Data will be recorded with a band-pass filter of 0.3–70 Hz and digitized at a sampling rate of 512 Hz and analog-digital precision was 16 bits (Gal-Nt, EbNeuro®, Florence, Italy). Horizontal and vertical eye movements will be detected by electrooculogram (EOG). Subjects will be sat in a reclined chair for approximately 20 min. Data will be collected at a sampling rate of 256 Hz, with a common mode rejection ratio of 105 dB (decibel), and the following band pass characteristics: 0.1 Hz high-pass filter, 100 Hz fifth order low-pass filter Diagnostic test: CSF collection and AD biomarker measurement • The CSF samples will be collected by lumbar puncture, immediately centrifuged, and stored at −80 °C until performing the analysis. Aβ42, Aβ42/Aβ40 ratio, t-tau, and p-tau will be measured using a chemiluminescent enzyme immunoassay (CLEIA) analyzer LUMIPULSE® G600 (Fujirebio, Tokyo, Japan) Diagnostic test: neuropsychological evaluation • For extensive neuropsychological evaluation the investigators will use the following tools: global measurements (MMSE, Information-Memory-Concentration Test), tasks exploring verbal and spatial short- and long-term memory (Digit Span, Corsi Tapping Test, Five Words and Paired Words Acquisition and Recall after 10 min and 24 h, Short Story Immediate and Delayed Recall), prospective memory (Rivermead Behavioral Memory Test), attention (Trail Making Test A, Dual Task), language (Token Test, naming pictures, Category Fluency Task, Phonemic Fluency Task), constructional praxis (Copying Drawings and Rey-Osterrieth complex figure) and executive function (Trail Making Test B, Stroop Test, Frontal Assessment Battery, Weigl Test) To assess independent living skills, the investigators will use two structured interviews: Activities of Daily Living Scale (ADL) and Instrumental Activities of Daily Living Scale (IADL) Diagnostic test: assessment of cognitive reserve, depression, personality traits and leisure activities • In order to estimate premorbid intelligence, all cases will perform TIB test (Test di Intelligenza Breve), an Italian version of the National Adult Reading Test (NART) To assess personality traits of the subjects, the investigators will use the Big Five Factors Questionnaire (BFFQ), that measures the five factors of emotional stability, energy, conscientiousness, agreeableness and openness to culture and experience For cognitive reserve. Subjects will perform structured interviewed regarding participation in intellectual, sporting and social activities, in the course of their life The presence of depressive symptoms will be evaluated by means of the 22-item Hamilton Depression Rating Scale (HDRS) Diagnostic test: clinical-neuropsychological follow-up • For follow-up assessment, each subject will perform a complete clinical evaluation, an extensive neuropsychological evaluation (27 test), assessment of independent living skills (ADL and IADL), estimation of premorbid intelligence (TIB test) and scale for depression (Hamilton Depression Rating Scale—HDRS) Diagnostic test: ERP recording • For ERP acquisition the same EEG system that was used for EEG data acquisition will be used. The participants will be administered an ERP test battery with concurrently recorded EEG consisting of a 3-choice vigilance task (3CVT) designed to evaluate sustained attention and standard image recognition memory task (SIR) designed to evaluate attention, encoding, and image recognition memory. In the SIR, images will be chosen as stimuli to distinguish short term from semantic memory loss and extend previous results of image recognition ERP effects

Group/cohort	Intervention/treatment
Patients with mild cognitive impairment Patients diagnosed with MCI	Genetic: genetic analysis of APOE and BDNF genes • The three SNPs (rs429358, rs7412, and rs6265 on APOE and BDNF genes, respectively) will be analyzed by the polymerase chain reaction (PCR) on genomic DNA and with the analysis of melting curves (HRMA) using the Rotor-Gene 6000 (Rotor-Gene, Corbett Research, Mortlake, Australia) Diagnostic test: EEG recording • The EEG activity will be recorded continuously from 19 sites by using electrodes set in an elastic cap and positioned according to the 10–20 international system. The recording will be referenced to the common average of all electrodes, excluding Fp1 and Fp2. Re-referencing will be done prior to the EEG artifact detection and analysis. Data will be recorded with a band-pass filter of 0.3–70 Hz and digitized at a sampling rate of 512 Hz and analog-digital precision was 16 bits (Gal-Nt, EbNeuro®, Florence, Italy). Horizontal and vertical eye movements will be detected by electrooculogram (EOG). Subjects will be sat in a reclined chair for approximately 20 min. Data will be collected at a sampling rate of 256 Hz, with a common mode rejection ratio of 105 dB (decibel), and the following band pass characteristics: 0.1 Hz high-pass filter, 100 Hz fifth-order low-pass filter Diagnostic test: CSF collection and AD biomarker measurement • The CSF samples will be collected by lumbar puncture, immediately centrifuged, and stored at −80 °C until performing the analysis. $A\beta42$, $A\beta42/A\beta40$ ratio, t-tau, and p-tau will be measured using a chemiluminescent enzyme immunoassay (CLEIA) analyzer LUMIPULSE® G600 (Fujirebio, Tokyo, Japan) Diagnostic test: neuropsychological evaluation • For extensive neuropsychological evaluation the investigators will use the following tools: global measurements (MMSE, Information-Memory-Concentration Test), tasks exploring verbal and spatial short- and long-term memory (Digit Span, Corsi Tapping Test, Five Words and Paired Words Acquisition and Recall after 10 min and 24 h, Short Story Immediate and Delayed Recall), prospective memory (Rivermead Behavioral Memory Test), attention (Trail Making Test A, Dual Task), language (Token Test, naming pictures, Category Fluency Task, Phonemic Fluency Task), constructional praxis (Copying Drawings and Rey-Osterrieth complex figure) and executive function (Trail Making Test B, Stroop Test, Frontal Assessment Battery, Weigl Test) To assess independent living skills, the investigators will use two structured interviews: Activities of Daily Living Scale (ADL) and Instrumental Activities of Daily Living Scale (IADL) Diagnostic test: assessment of cognitive reserve, depression, personality traits and leisure activities • In order to estimate premorbid intelligence, all cases will perform TIB test (Test di Intelligenza Breve), an Italian version of the National Adult Reading Test (NART). To assess personality traits of the subjects, the investigators will use the Big Five Factors Questionnaire (BFFQ), that measures the five factors of emotional stability, energy, conscientiousness, agreeableness and openness to culture and experience For cognitive reserve. Subjects will perform structured interviewed regarding participation in intellectual, sporting and social activities, in the course of their life The presence of depressive symptoms will be evaluated by means of the 22-item Hamilton Depression Rating Scale (HDRS) Diagnostic test: clinical-neuropsychological follow-up • For follow-up assessment, each subject will perform a complete clinical evaluation, an extensive neuropsychological evaluation (27 test), assessment of independent living skills (ADL and IADL), estimation of premorbid intelligence (TIB test) and scale for depression (Hamilton Depression Rating Scale—HDRS) Diagnostic test: ERP recording • For ERP acquisition the same EEG system that was used for EEG data acquisition will be used. The participants will be administered an ERP test battery with concurrently recorded EEG consisting of a 3-choice vigilance task (3CVT) designed to evaluate sustained attention and standard image recognition memory task (SIR) designed to evaluate attention, encoding, and image recognition memory. In the SIR, images will be chosen as stimuli to distinguish short term from semantic memory loss and extend previous results of image recognition ERP effects

Group/cohort	Intervention/treatment
Healthy controls	Diagnostic test: EEG recording • The EEG activity will be recorded continuously from 19 sites by using electrodes set in an elastic cap and positioned according to the 10–20 international system. The recording will be referenced to the common average of all electrodes, excluding Fp1 and Fp2. Re-referencing will be done prior to the EEG artifact detection and analysis. Data will be recorded with a band-pass filter of 0.3–70 Hz and digitized at a sampling rate of 512 Hz and analog-digital precision was 16 bits (Gal-Nt, EbNeuro®, Florence, Italy). Horizontal and vertical eye movements will be detected by electrooculogram (EOG). Subjects will be sat in a reclined chair for approximately 20 min. Data will be collected at a sampling rate of 256 Hz, with a common mode rejection ratio of 105 dB (decibel), and the following band pass characteristics: 0.1 Hz high-pass filter, 100 Hz fifth order low-pass filter Diagnostic test: ERP recording • For ERP acquisition, the same EEG system that was used for EEG data acquisition will be used. The participants will be administered an ERP test battery with concurrently recorded EEG consisting of a 3-choice vigilance task (3CVT) designed to evaluate sustained attention and a standard image recognition memory task (SIR) designed to evaluate attention, encoding, and image recognition memory. In the SIR, images will be chosen as stimuli to distinguish short term from semantic memory loss and extend previous results of image recognition ERP effects

Primary outcome measures

Outcome measure	Measure description	Time frame
Clinical diagnosis of MCI in patients diagnosed with SCD	Patients diagnosed with SCD at baseline will be followed up every 6 months by neurological evaluation and every 12 months by neuropsychological examination in order to detect progression to MCI according to National Institute on Aging and Alzheimer's Association (NIA-AA) criteria	3 years
Clinical diagnosis of AD in patients diagnosed with SCD and MCI	Patients diagnosed with SCD or MCI at baseline will be followed up every 6 months by neurological evaluation and every 12 months by neuropsychological examination in order to detect progression to AD according to NIA-AA criteria	3 years

Secondary outcome measures

Outcome measure	Measure description	Time frame
Variations in neuropsychological scores	All included patients will be evaluated every 12 months by extensive neuropsychological examinations in order to identify variations in cognitive performances	2 years

Sponsor

Azienda Ospedaliero-Universitaria Careggi

Collaborators

- Fondazione Don Carlo Gnocchi Onlus
- University of Florence
- Scuola Superiore Sant'Anna di Pisa

Investigators

- Principal Investigator:Valentina Bessi, MD, PhD, Research and Innovation Centre for Dementia-CRIDEM, AOU Careggi, Florence, Italy

General Publications

- Giacomucci G, Mazzeo S, Bagnoli S, Casini M, Padiglioni S, Polito C, Berti V, Balestrini J, Ferrari C, Lombardi G, Ingannato A, Sorbi S, Nacmias B, Bessi V. Matching Clinical Diagnosis and Amyloid Biomarkers in Alzheimer's Disease and Frontotemporal Dementia. J Pers Med. 2021 Jan 14;11(1):47. https://doi.org/10.3390/jpm11010047.
- Mazzeo S, Bessi V, Bagnoli S, Giacomucci G, Balestrini J, Padiglioni S, Tomaiuolo G, Ingannato A, Ferrari C, Bracco L, Sorbi S, Nacmias B. Dual Effect of PER2 C111G Polymorphism on Cognitive Functions across Progression from Subjective Cognitive Decline to Mild Cognitive Impairment. Diagnostics (Basel). 2021 Apr 18;11(4):718. https://doi.org/10.3390/diagnostics11040718.
- Bessi V, Balestrini J, Bagnoli S, Mazzeo S, Giacomucci G, Padiglioni S, Piaceri I, Carraro M, Ferrari C, Bracco L, Sorbi S, Nacmias B. Influence of ApoE Genotype and Clock T3111C Interaction with Cardiovascular Risk Factors on the Progression to Alzheimer's Disease in Subjective Cognitive Decline and Mild Cognitive Impairment Patients. J Pers Med. 2020 May 29;10(2):45. https://doi.org/10.3390/jpm10020045.
- Mazzeo S, Padiglioni S, Bagnoli S, Bracco L, Nacmias B, Sorbi S, Bessi V. The dual role of cognitive reserve in subjective cognitive decline and mild cognitive impairment: a 7-year follow-up study. J Neurol. 2019 Feb;266(2):487–497. https://doi.org/10.1007/s00415-018-9164-5. Epub 2019 Jan 2.
- Giacomucci G, Mazzeo S, Padiglioni S, Bagnoli S, Belloni L, Ferrari C, Bracco L, Nacmias B, Sorbi S, Bessi V. Gender differences in cognitive reserve: implication for subjective cognitive decline in women. Neurol Sci. 2022 Apr;43(4):2499–2508. https://doi.org/10.1007/s10072-021-05644-x. Epub 2021 Oct 8.
- Mazzeo S, Bessi V, Padiglioni S, Bagnoli S, Bracco L, Sorbi S, Nacmias B. KIBRA T allele influences memory performance and progression of cognitive decline: a 7-year follow-up study in subjective cognitive decline and mild cognitive impairment. Neurol Sci. 2019 Aug;40(8):1559–1566. https://doi.org/10.1007/s10072-019-03866-8. Epub 2019 Apr 5.
- Bessi V, Mazzeo S, Padiglioni S, Piccini C, Nacmias B, Sorbi S, Bracco L. From Subjective Cognitive Decline to Alzheimer's Disease: The Predictive Role of Neuropsychological Assessment, Personality Traits, and Cognitive Reserve. A 7-Year Follow-Up Study. J Alzheimers Dis. 2018;63(4):1523–1535. https://doi.org/10.3233/JAD-171180.
- Mazzeo S, Padiglioni S, Bagnoli S, Carraro M, Piaceri I, Bracco L, Nacmias B, Sorbi S, Bessi V. Assessing the effectiveness of subjective cognitive decline plus criteria in predicting the progression to Alzheimer's disease: an 11-year follow-up study. Eur J Neurol. 2020 May;27(5):894–899. https://doi.org/10.1111/ene.14167. Epub 2020 Mar 8.
- Amoroso N, Diacono D, Fanizzi A, La Rocca M, Monaco A, Lombardi A, Guaragnella C, Bellotti R, Tangaro S; Alzheimer's Disease Neuroimaging Initiative. Deep learning reveals Alzheimer's disease onset in MCI subjects: Results from an international challenge. J Neurosci Methods. 2018 May 15;302:3–9. https://doi.org/10.1016/j.jneumeth.2017.12.011. Epub 2017 Dec 26.

- Bansal D. et al. Comparative Analysis of Various Machine Learning Algorithms for Detecting Dementia—Procedia Computer Science (2018) 132:1497–1502
- Gouw AA, Alsema AM, Tijms BM, Borta A, Scheltens P, Stam CJ, van der Flier WM. EEG spectral analysis as a putative early prognostic biomarker in nondemented, amyloid positive subjects. Neurobiol Aging. 2017 Sep;57:133–142. https://doi.org/10.1016/j.neurobiolaging.2017.05.017. Epub 2017 Jun 1.
- Guillem F, Rougier A, Claverie B. Short- and long-delay intracranial ERP repetition effects dissociate memory systems in the human brain. J Cogn Neurosci. 1999 Jul;11(4):437–58. https://doi.org/10.1162/089892999563526.

EEG/ERP

Recruiting

United States

Event-Related Potential (ERP) Components in Clinical Diagnosis

ClinicalTrials.gov ID NCT05673759

Sponsor Boston University
Information provided by Boston University (Responsible Party)
Last Update Posted 2023-03-28

Study Overview

Brief Summary

In this study, the investigators will use a novel electroencephalogram (EEG) system that participants will wear during a single in-person research session to investigate whether ERPs are now ready for validation as a tool clinicians can easily implement to increase diagnostic accuracy and confidence. This EEG will not be used to treat, cure, mitigate, or diagnose any disease and there will be no safety or efficacy data collected about the machine for any purpose including support of FDA submission.

The investigators will compare the ERP data to that of neuropsychological testing in order to determine the degree of correlation between these two measures. Questionnaires on cognition, mood, and fluency will be administered prior to the EEG to establish a baseline. ERP data from the EEG session will be compared with the results of the neuropsychological battery in order to determine whether the implementation of ERPs in the existing workflow of clinicians can aid in diagnostic accuracy, thus altering clinical management.

Detailed Description

A cross-sectional cohort study design with four groups will be implemented to determine how ERPs can provide diagnostic information and alter clinical management beyond that of neuropsychological testing alone in patients with Alzheimer's disease (AD) or Mild Cognitive Impairment (MCI).

Secondary Objectives
- To determine the impact of ERP testing (using cognitive health assessment reports) on change in research grade clinical diagnosis.
- To determine the degree of correlation between quantitative ERP measures with neuropsychological testing performance using a standardized neuropsychological battery.

Seventy-five mild AD dementia and 75 MCI due to any etiology, 25 Older Adults (OA), and 25 Younger Adults (YA) will be enrolled over the course of 2 years. Each subject will participate in the study for 1 visit.

The in-person 50–60-min testing session consists of a neuropsychological battery, and an EEG session with computer tasks including the Auditory Oddball paradigm, a Continuous Visual Memory Test, Auditory-Evoked Potentials, Visual-Evoked Potentials, the Erikson Flanker Task, and the Hayling Task.

Official Title
The Clinical Utility of ERPs in the Diagnosis of Cognitive Impairment

Conditions
Alzheimer Disease
Dementia, Mild
Mild Cognitive Impairment

Intervention/Treatment
- Device: Electroencephalogram (EEG) system
- Behavioral: Standard Neuropsychological Testing
- Behavioral: Additional neuropsychological tests

Other Study ID Numbers
- H-43360

Study Start (Actual)
2023-03-06

Primary Completion (Estimated)
2024-09

Study Completion (Estimated)
2024-09

Enrollment (Estimated)
200

Study Type
Observational

Study Contact
Name: Katherine Turk, MD
Phone Number: (617) 638-7730
Email: kturk@bu.edu

Study Contact Backup
Name: Meltem Karaca, PhD
Phone Number: (857) 364-2139
Email: mkaraca@bu.edu

United States
Massachusetts Locations

Boston, Massachusetts, United States, 02118
Recruiting
BU Alzheimer Disease Center

Contact
Meltem Karaca, PhD
mkaraca@bu.edu

Inclusion Criteria
For Mild Alzheimer Disease (AD) dementia

- Meets probable AD dementia National Institute on Aging and Alzheimer's Association (NIA-AA) criteria
- 50–90 years old
- Mini-Mental State Examination (MMSE) 20–27
- Performance on delayed recall and recognition memory worse than 1.5 standard deviations (SD) for age and education
- Performance on delayed recall and recognition memory worse than 1.5 SD for age and education in at least one other cognitive domain (e.g., language, executive functioning) based on other tests in our neuropsychological test battery
- Dr. Turk and Dr. Budson will confirm all mild AD dementia diagnoses

For mild cognitive impairment (MCI)

- MCI due to any etiology 50–90 years old
- MMSE >23
- Performance on delayed recall and recognition memory worse than 1.0 SD for age- and education-adjusted norms
- Dr. Turk and Dr. Budson will confirm all MCI diagnoses

For Healthy older adults

- 50–90 years old
- Functioning normally in occupation determined by self-report

For Healthy younger adults

- 20–50 years old
- Functioning normally in occupation determined by self-report

Exclusion Criteria
- A clinically significant problem of any of the following conditions:
- depression

- heavy alcohol or drug use
- cerebrovascular disease
- a different degenerative disease (e.g., fronto-temporal dementia, Parkinson's disease)
- any medical condition whose severity could significantly impair cognition (e.g., organ failure)
- on any antipsychotic or epilepsy medication
- unable to understand the consent form

Study Population

Any participant age: 20–90 years old, with or without a diagnosis of AD or cognitive impairment.

Ages Eligible for Study

20 Years to 90 Years (Adult, Older Adult)

Sexes Eligible for Study

All

Accepts Healthy Volunteers

Yes

Sampling Method

Probability Sample

Design Details

Observational Model: Cohort
Time Perspective: Cross-Sectional

Cohorts and interventions

Group/cohort	Intervention/treatment

75 Mild AD
75 patients diagnosed with Mild Alzheimer's disease
	Device: Electroencephalogram (EEG) system
	• An FDA 510(k) approved EEG/ERP device designed by G-Tec™ intended for the acquisition, display, analysis, storage, reporting, and management of EEG and auditory-evoked potentials (AEP) information and uses Bluetooth technology to securely transmit EEG signals to a computer. The device is patient-friendly, and no serious adverse events have occurred to date in any research or clinical study or in clinical use
	• Other names:
	  – g.Nautilus PRO (G-Tec™)
	Behavioral: Standard Neuropsychological Testing
	• Prior to the EEG session, neuropsychological testing will be done to establish a baseline measurement. We administer a full standard neuropsychological battery (45 min) for all participants which includes the following tests: MOCA (only for older participants), MMSE, CERAD, Phonemic Test and the Category Fluency test, Trails Making Test A and B, BNT, BAI, BDI, PANAS, Ishihara Color Blindness test, and the Snellen Eye Chart
	• Other names:
	  – Neuropsychological Battery

Group/cohort	Intervention/treatment

75 MCI due to any etiology 75 patients diagnosed with Mild Cognitive Impairment due to any etiology	Device: Electroencephalogram (EEG) system
	• An FDA 510(k) approved EEG/ERP device designed by G-Tec™ intended for the acquisition, display, analysis, storage, reporting, and management of EEG and auditory-evoked potentials (AEP) information and uses Bluetooth technology to securely transmit EEG signals to a computer. The device is patient-friendly, and no serious adverse events have occurred to date in any research or clinical study or in clinical use
	• Other names:
	  – e.g. Nautilus PRO (G-Tec™)
	Behavioral: Standard Neuropsychological Testing
	• Prior to the EEG session, neuropsychological testing will be done to establish a baseline measurement. We administer a full standard neuropsychological battery (45 min) for all participants which includes the following tests: MOCA (only for older participants), MMSE, CERAD, Phonemic Test and the Category Fluency test, Trails Making Test A and B, BNT, BAI, BDI, PANAS, Ishihara Color Blindness test, and the Snellen Eye Chart
	• Other names:
	  – Neuropsychological Battery

25 Healthy Older Adults 25 Healthy Older Adults age: 50–90 (control)	Device: Electroencephalogram (EEG) system
	• An FDA 510(k) approved EEG/ERP device designed by G-Tec™ intended for the acquisition, display, analysis, storage, reporting, and management of EEG and auditory-evoked potentials (AEP) information and uses Bluetooth technology to securely transmit EEG signals to a computer. The device is patient-friendly, and no serious adverse events have occurred to date in any research or clinical study or in clinical use
	• Other names:
	  – e.g., Nautilus PRO (G-Tec™)
	Behavioral: Standard Neuropsychological Testing
	• Prior to the EEG session, neuropsychological testing will be done to establish a baseline measurement. We administer a full standard neuropsychological battery (45 min) for all participants which includes the following tests: MOCA (only for older participants), MMSE, CERAD, Phonemic Test and the Category Fluency test, Trails Making Test A and B, BNT, BAI, BDI, PANAS, Ishihara Color Blindness test, and the Snellen Eye Chart.
	• Other names:
	  – Neuropsychological Battery

Group/cohort	Intervention/treatment

25 Healthy Younger Adults
25 Healthy Younger Adults age: 20–50 (control)
	Device: Electroencephalogram (EEG) system
	• An FDA 510(k) approved EEG/ERP device designed by G-Tec™ intended for the acquisition, display, analysis, storage, reporting, and management of EEG and auditory-evoked potentials (AEP) information and uses Bluetooth technology to securely transmit EEG signals to a computer. The device is patient-friendly, and no serious adverse events have occurred to date in any research or clinical study or in clinical use
	• Other names:
	  – g.Nautilus PRO (G-Tec™)
	Behavioral: Standard Neuropsychological Testing
	• Prior to the EEG session, neuropsychological testing will be done to establish a baseline measurement. We administer a full standard neuropsychological battery (45 min) for all participants which includes the following tests: MOCA (only for older participants), MMSE, CERAD, Phonemic Test and the Category Fluency test, Trails Making Test A and B, BNT, BAI, BDI, PANAS, Ishihara Color Blindness test, and the Snellen Eye Chart
	• Other names:
	  – Neuropsychological Battery
	Behavioral: additional neuropsychological tests
	• Younger participants will receive additional testing along with the standard neuropsychological battery including Pittsburgh Sleep Quality Index (PSQI) for sleep quality measures, the Test of Memory Malingering (TOMM) for effort measure, Ohio State Traumatic Brain Injury Identification Method questionnaire (OSU-TBI) to gather lifetime TBI history, and the Neurobehavioral Symptom Inventory (NBSI) for post-concussive symptoms. These additional tests will add an extra 15 min, making the total time for neuropsychological questionnaires 1 h in younger participants

Primary outcome measures

Outcome measure	Measure description	Time frame
Electroencephalogram (EEG) memory diagnosis	The EEG memory diagnosis will be arrived at through the blinded review of the EEG data	Baseline

Secondary outcome measures

Outcome measure	Measure description	Time frame
The Montreal Cognitive Assessment (MoCA) performance	This neuropsychological test will be used for cognitive screening. The scores on this test range from 0 to 30, and lower scores indicate decreased cognitive ability	Baseline
Mini Mental State Examination (MMSE)	This neuropsychological test will be used to assess cognitive functioning. MMSE scores range from 0 to 30 with lower scores indicating decreased cognitive ability	Baseline

Outcome measure	Measure description	Time frame
Consortium to Establish a Registry in Alzheimer's disease Word List Test (CERAD)	The CERAD evaluates the immediate recall of a list of words (up to 30 correct recall on 3 individual recall trials), delayed recall (up to 10 correct recall after a 5 min delay), and on yes–no recognition memory (up to 10 correct recognition)	Baseline
Verbal Fluency test: Phonemic Test and the Category Fluency test	Phonemic word fluency and categoric word fluency will be assessed using the Verbal Fluency: Phonemic Test and the Category Fluency test. For letter fluency, individuals name as many words as possible in 1 min that start with the letters F, A, and S. For category fluency, individuals name as many words as possible in 1 min that are within the Animals, Vegetables, and Fruits categories	Baseline
Trails Making Test A and B	The Trail Making Test Part A consists of connecting a series of numbers with a line in ascending order as quickly as possible (performance is timed and the score is the time to complete the task). The Trail Making Test Part B consists of connecting a series of letters and numbers, alternating back and forth between them, as quickly as possible in ascending order (performance is timed, and the score is the time to complete). The test will be used to assess the central executive functioning	Baseline
Boston Naming Test	This test consists of 15 line drawings, with a maximum score of 15 correct. It will be used to assess naming skills in speakers of multiple languages	Baseline
EEG amplitude	EEG amplitudes will be measured from the EEG data	Baseline
EEG latency	EEG latency will be measured from the EEG data	Baseline

Sponsor

Boston University

Collaborators

- VoxNeuro Inc.

Investigators

- Principal Investigator: Katherine Turk, MD, BU Chobanian & Avedisian School of Medicine
- Principal Investigator: Andrew Budson, MD, BU Chobanian & Avedisian School of Medicine

General Publications

No publications available

Eye Tracking

Recruiting

Canada

Development and Validation of a Novel Functional Eye-Tracking Software Application for Alzheimer's Disease

ClinicalTrials.gov ID NCT05176704

Sponsor Innodem Neurosciences
Information provided by Innodem Neurosciences (Responsible Party)
Last Update Posted 2022-09-22

Brief Summary

This study aims to develop and validate a sensitive and noninvasive eye-tracking software application.

This study will obtain participant responses to brief cognitive tests designed to evaluate several key functions known to be affected by Alzheimer's Disease and noninvasive eye movement measurements in response to visually presented stimuli during specifically designed eye-tracking tests. The study data will be used to develop machine learning algorithms and validate a software application intended to track the progressive component of Alzheimer's Disease and associated cognitive changes.

Official Title

Development and Validation of a Novel Functional Eye-Tracking Software Application for Alzheimer's Disease

Conditions

Alzheimer's Disease

Intervention/Treatment

- Device: Eye-Tracking

Other Study ID Numbers

- ETNA-AD

Study Start (Actual)

2022-04-15

Primary Completion (Estimated)

2023-11-30

Study Completion (Estimated)

2023-11-30

Enrollment (Estimated)
250

Study Type
Observational [Patient Registry]

Study Contact
Name: Nancy Mugisha
Phone Number: (514) 761-6131 ext 3451
Email: nancy.mugisha.comtl@ssss.gouv.qc.ca
Canada
Quebec Locations

Montréal, Quebec, Canada, H4H 1R3
Recruiting
The Douglas Research Centre

Contact
Nancy Mugisha
(514) 761-6131 ext 3451 nancy.mugisha.comtl@ssss.gouv.qc.ca

Principal Investigator
Simon Ducharme

Inclusion Criteria
- For all participants:

  - Able to provide informed consent
  - Aged 18 years or older at the time of enrollment
  - Able to read in either French or English
  - Visual acuity of 20/100 in at least one eye (corrective glasses, contact lenses, surgery, etc. are permitted)

- For patients only:

  - Confirmed diagnosis of AD based on the NIAAA diagnostic criteria of probable AD
  - Having undergone a full neuropsychological evaluation within the last 6 months or having a planned full neuropsychological evaluation within the next 6 months.
  - AD diagnoses supported by FDG-PET scan or amyloid biomarkers (CSF or amyloid PET)

Exclusion Criteria
- For AD participants:

  - Diagnosed with one of the following dementia subtypes: Fronto-temporal dementia, Lewy-body dementia, or Creutzfeldt–Jakob disease.
  - Incapacity to provide informed consent or inability to adequately understand the task instructions.

- For all participants:

  - Evidence or medical history of psychiatric issues, which are known to also affect movements and oculomotor control.
  - Presence of comorbid neurological conditions to avoid eye movement anomaly confounds (strabismus, cranial nerve palsy, stroke-causing hemianopsia).
  - Diagnosis of macular edema or other pre-existing ocular conditions (e.g., glaucoma, cataracts) that would prevent from performing the eye movement assessments.
  - Unstable medication use: recent (less than 1 month from enrollment) start of, change of dose, or irregular use of, new prescription drugs known to have an effect on ocular motor visual function, such as benzodiazepines, antipsychotics, and anticonvulsants. Occasional use of benzodiazepines for medical procedures is permitted, at the investigator's discretion, but should not occur within a short time period of an eye movement assessment.
  - Diagnosed with an active substance use disorder.
  - History of stroke.
  - Recent traumatic brain injury (within the last 6 months).

- For healthy controls only:

  - Evidence or history of significant neurodegenerative disorder affecting brain function (e.g., MS, PD, ALS, Non-AD Dementia)

Study Population

For this study, we will recruit 250 participants. Two hundred will be AD patients (including predominant AD with mixed vascular and MCI due to AD), who will subsequently be divided into 4 sub-groups of 50 based on their CDR score (questionable/very mild dementia (CDR = 0.5), mild dementia/MCI (CDR = 1), moderate dementia (CDR = 2), and severe dementia (CDR = 3)), and 50 will be healthy cognitively intact age-matched control participants.

Ages Eligible for Study

18 Years and older (Adult, Older Adult)

Sexes Eligible for Study

All

Accepts Healthy Volunteers

Yes

Sampling Method

Probability Sample

Design Details

Observational Model: Cohort
Time Perspective: Cross-Sectional
Target Follow-up Duration: 1 Day

Cohorts and interventions

Group/cohort	Intervention/treatment
CDR = 0.5 50 Alzheimer's disease (AD) patients including predominant AD with mixed vascular and MCI due to AD based on their CDR score. Questionable/very mild dementia (CDR = 0.5)	Device: eye-tracking • Eye-tracking technology and algorithms used to successfully capture and track eye movements using an electronic tablet and the embedded camera of the device
CDR = 1 50 Alzheimer's disease (AD) patients including predominant AD with mixed vascular and MCI due to AD based on their CDR score. Mild dementia/MCI (CDR = 1)	Device: eye-tracking • Eye-tracking technology and algorithms used to successfully capture and track eye movements using an electronic tablet and the embedded camera of the device
CDR = 2 50 Alzheimer's disease (AD) patients including predominant AD with mixed vascular and MCI due to AD based on their CDR score. Moderate dementia (CDR = 2)	Device: eye-tracking • Eye-tracking technology and algorithms used to successfully capture and track eye movements using an electronic tablet and the embedded camera of the device
CDR = 3 50 Alzheimer's disease (AD) patients including predominant AD with mixed vascular and MCI due to AD based on their CDR score. Severe dementia (CDR = 3)	Device: eye-tracking • Eye-tracking technology and algorithms used to successfully capture and track eye movements using an electronic tablet and the embedded camera of the device
Healthy control Fifty participants with no evidence or history of significant neurodegenerative disorder affecting brain function	Device: eye-tracking • Eye-tracking technology and algorithms used to successfully capture and track eye movements using an electronic tablet and the embedded camera of the device

Primary outcome measures

Outcome measure	Measure description	Time frame
Clinical Dementia Rating (CDR) score, one time, on the day of enrollment	The Clinical Dementia Rating (CDR) is a global rating scale for staging patients diagnosed with Alzheimer's disease and other dementias and monitoring changes in the level of their disabilities over time. The CDR scale is a 0–3 point numeric scale (0.5 unit increments) derived from clinician rating of cognition and daily function in the domains of memory, orientation, judgment and problem-solving, community affairs, home and hobbies, and personal care	Baseline

Secondary outcome measures

Outcome measure	Measure description	Time frame
The Montreal Cognitive Assessment (MoCA) score, one time, on the day of enrollment	The Montreal Cognitive Assessment (MoCA) is a brief 30-question cognitive screening test designed to assist Health Professionals in the detection of mild cognitive impairment and Alzheimer's disease. It assesses different cognitive domains: attention and concentration, executive functions, memory, language, visuoconstructional skills, conceptual thinking, calculations, and orientation. Scores on the MoCA range from 0 to 30, with a score of 26 and higher generally considered normal	Baseline
The Mini-Mental State Exam (MMSE) score, one time, on the day of enrollment	The Mini-Mental State Exam (MMSE) is a widely used test of cognitive function among the elderly, it includes tests of orientation, attention, memory, language, and visual-spatial skills. It consists of a series of questions and tests that can be used by clinicians to help diagnose dementia and to help assess its progression and severity	Baseline

Sponsor

Innodem Neurosciences

Collaborators

No information provided

Investigators

No information provided

General Publications

No publications available

Eye Tracking

Recruiting

Canada

BEAM: Brain-Eye Amyloid Memory Study (BEAM)

ClinicalTrials.gov ID NCT02524405

Sponsor Sunnybrook Health Sciences Centre
Information provided by Dr. Sandra E Black, Sunnybrook Health Sciences Centre (Responsible Party)
Last Update Posted 2022-10-25

Brief Summary

The main objectives of this study are:

1. To investigate novel, noninvasive ocular measurements including optical coherence tomography and eye tracking in a cross-sectional study of participants with various neurodegenerative dementias against standard cognitive assessments and brain imaging measures.
2. To assess the potential utility of ocular assessments for early detection in the pre-dementia, i.e., the so-called Mild Cognitive Impairment (MCI) stage, across the common neurodegenerative dementia syndromes and, Vascular Cognitive Impairment (VCI) due to small vessel disease (SVD).
3. To determine the prevalence and relevance of amyloid uptake on PET scanning across the dementias most commonly associated with amyloidosis. Specifically, we aim to examine correlations with amyloid uptake status in patients symptomatic from the most common proteinopathies (i.e., amyloid, tau, synuclein) combined in varying degrees with the most common vasculopathies (i.e., small vessel disease) using multimodal structural and functional imaging, cognitive behavioral, and gait and balance measures, taking into account genetic risk markers (particularly apolipoprotein E genotypes) and fluid biomarkers (e.g., cytokines, oxidative stress, lipidomics).

Detailed Description

1. Retinal correlations with neurodegeneration:

   (a) Retinal nerve fiber layer (RNFL) pattern will differ in participants in the MCI and early stages of LBD spectrum, AD, and VCI, relative to normal elders. (a) RNFL thinning around the optic disc and macular thinning will correlate with hippocampal atrophy and with the cortical thickness signature of MCI and AD2-4. (b) If detected in the other disorders, RNFL thinning will also correlate with this topographical AD pattern of atrophy in those who are amyloid positive on PET. (c) Retinal and cortical thinning will predict brain amyloid PET. (d) Selective peripapillary RNFL thinning in the superior and inferior quadrants described in MCI/milder AD cases will correlate with precuneus and lingual gyrus cortical thinning, respectively.

   (b) Retinal artery narrowing will correlate with the presence of covert lacunar infarcts and retinal venular widening with moderate to severe periventricular white matter hyperintensities.

2. Amyloid deposition above accepted cut-offs will vary across the four cohorts and when present will correlate meaningfully with cognitive and behavioral patterns, including ocular (retinal and eye tracking), gait and balance measures, and brain imaging results.

Specific hypotheses are:

1. Apolipoprotein E e4 carrier status will increase the likelihood of amyloid positivity across the cohorts.

2. Amyloid positivity will be associated with poorer short-term memory performance, smaller hippocampal volumes, greater cortical thinning in signature
   areas traditionally associated with Alzheimer's disease, and also with lobar
   microbleed counts.
3. Small Vessel Disease burden as quantified on PD/T2 and FLAIR MRI will be
   associated with speed of processing, attention, and executive functions and with
   a different pattern of cortical thinning involving more inferior and medial frontal
   regions.
4. Amyloid deposition as measured by the regional standardized uptake value ratio
   (SUVR), and Small Vessel Disease burden will correlate differentially with
   structural imaging measures, as well as both functional and structural brain connectivity measures.

Study Procedures Overview. The study procedures are listed below in the recom-
mended order of assessment but may be performed in any sequence (with specific
exceptions as described). Multiple assessments may be performed on the same day
for participant convenience. Brain imaging and neuropsychology procedures should
be completed within 4 months of screening.

Screening Visit Consent. The study will be explained and written informed consent for participation will be obtained from the patient or his/her substitute decision
maker and the participant's study partner (if applicable).

Screening. The general and disease-specific inclusion and exclusion criteria will
be assessed. If the MMSE, MoCA, DOC (Depression, Obstructive Sleep Apnea,
Cognition) questionnaire, and/or TorCA (formally known as Behavioural Neurology
Assessment-Revised) (BNA-R) have not been administered within the past 4
months, they will be administered at the screening visit. Information on the patient's
concomitant medications, medical, surgical, ophthalmological history, family health
history, and other relevant history will be collected, as well as information on both
the patient's and the study partner's demographics. The patient's corrected near
visual acuity will be checked. Auditory acuity at various frequencies will be assessed
using an audiometer. Fasting blood will be drawn, for the analysis of HbA1c, CBC,
electrolytes, creatinine, urea, lipid profile, glucose, liver function (AST, ALT, ALP,
bilirubin), homocysteine, B12, and TSH. Blood will also be drawn for genomics
and fluid biomarkers (see next section).

Genomics and Fluid Biomarkers. Fasting blood samples for genetic testing,
including apolipoprotein E4 status, as well as for proteomic, lipidomic, and other
fluid biomarkers of neurodegeneration and vascular disease, will be collected from
each participant.

Neuropsychological Battery and Questionnaires. The cognitive battery com-
prises most of the tests used in the Ontario Neurodegenerative Disease Research
Initiative (ONDRI) study, a new province-wide neurodegeneration research collab-
oration, with some modifications. It includes measures of executive function, memory, language, and visuospatial ability. Function, mood, behavior, and caregiver
burden will also be assessed using the questionnaires used in ONDRI. The full list
of the assessment procedures is included in the BEAM neuropsychology manuals.

SD-OCT. Assessments to meet ocular criteria will include visual acuity, intra-ocular pressure (IOP) measurement, and a nonmydriatic fundus camera recording, performed by a certified ophthalmic technician. The participant will then undergo SD-OCT to determine retinal nerve fiber layer thickness.

Vital Signs and Neurological Exam. Vital signs will be measured and a neurological examination will be performed.

Gait and Balance Assessment. Information on aid use and balance will be collected using questionnaires. Participants' leg length, calf circumference, height, and weight will be measured and recorded when possible.

Eye Tracking. Participants will be asked to look at a computer monitor and perform three sets of tasks (pro-saccade, anti-saccade, and dynamic free viewing) while a specialized camera tracks and records their eye movements. Participants who are unable to complete these assessments will be allowed to continue participation in the study.

SV-OCT at Sunnybrook. SV-OCT will be done in subsamples with high SVD vs. minimal SVD loads. A rapid (>100 fps) 3D scanning protocol will be applied to SD-OCT, allowing the acquisition of speckle variance due to microscopic blood flow in the retinal vasculature. Image processing using GPU-based technique will provide real-time assessment of microvasculature morphology.

MRI. 3DT1 SPGR, interleaved spin echo PD/T2, and FLAIR to assess SVD, and gradient echo images to assess microbleeds will be obtained on the 3 T scanners at each of the TDRA sites. The PD/T2 and FLAIR images are co-registered to the T1-weighted image to remove nonbrain tissues to determine the total supratentorial intracranial volume to correct for head size, classify brain tissue compartments, and automatically identify subcortical and white matter hyperintensities using a published in-house pipeline, "Lesion Explorer," which with manual editing yields number, size, location, and volume of the hyperintensities. For hippocampal volume, we use our fully automated segmentation pipeline based on a template library registration. We will also acquire DTI to generate total and regional fractional anisotropy (FA) and Mean Diffusivity Maps, using FSL and DTI toolbox, and a resting state fMRI to explore Default Mode Network (DMN) connectivity, using a processing pipeline steps previously applied to AD patients and controls.

Arterial Spin Labeling (ASL) will be included at certain sites which are capable of acquiring this sequence to obtain measures of regional cerebral perfusion.

Amyloid PET. PIB, labeled with the positron-emitting atom carbon-11, is a radiotracer that targets Aβ-aggregates (β-amyloid) in vivo. β-Amyloid deposits are present in the brains of patients with Alzheimer's disease (AD). Therefore, Aβ-plaques in the brain may be a useful biomarker of the disease and its progression and [11C]-PIB may be a useful tool to detect these plaques in the human living brain with PET.

[11C]-PIB is an investigational positron-emitting radiopharmaceutical (PER) not yet marketed in Canada. The ligand will be manufactured at the CAMH PET Centre. PET imaging will be performed using [11C] PIB at the CAMH PET Centre with PET/CT-Discovery MI scanner using the standardized acquisition protocol.

The PET imaging protocol begins with a low-dose CT scan (less than 0.05 mSv) for attenuation correction. Immediately following this acquisition, a bolus containing approximately 10 ± 1 mCi of [11C]-PIB is administered by IV injection, followed by 90 min acquisition. Acquisition and reconstruction of PET images are done according to the standard PET Centre Imaging Protocols.

Phone Check Ups: For safety measures, the participants will be contacted by phone to discuss any possible adverse event and general well-being two times during the course of the study:

- 24–72 h after the PET scan
- 30 days (+/− 7 days) after PET Scan and/or the last study procedure

Official Title

The Brain Eye Amyloid Memory (BEAM) Study: Validation of Ocular Measures as Potential Biomarkers for Early Detection of Brain Amyloid and Neurodegeneration

Conditions

Alzheimer's Disease
Mild Cognitive Impairment
Vascular Cognitive Impairment
Parkinson's Disease
Lewy Body Disease

Intervention/Treatment

- Other: Pittsburgh Compound B [11C]-PIB

Other Study ID Numbers

- 221-2013

Study Start

2016-02

Primary Completion (Estimated)

2024-03

Study Completion (Estimated)

2024-12

Enrollment (Estimated)

345

Study Type

Observational

Study Contact

Name: Sandra E Black, MD
Email: sandra.black@sunnybrook.ca
Canada
Ontario Locations

Toronto, Ontario, Canada, M4N 3 M5
Recruiting
Sunnybrook Health Sciences Centre

Contact
BSc

Principal Investigator
Sandra Black, MD

Toronto, Ontario, Canada, M5B 1W8
Recruiting
St. Michael's Hospital

Principal Investigator
Corinne Fischer, MD

Toronto, Ontario, Canada, M5T2S8
Recruiting
University Health Network

Principal Investigator
Carmela Tartaglia, MD, FRCPC

Toronto, Ontario, Canada, M6A 2E1
Recruiting
Baycrest Health Sciences

Contact
Brad Pugh
406.785.2500 ext 6207 b.pugh@baycrest.org

Principal Investigator
Morris Freedman, MD

Description

General Inclusion Criteria (All Subgroups)
Participants must meet each of the following criteria for enrolment into the study:

- Written informed consent obtained and documented
- Male or post-menopausal female (minimum of 1 year since the last menstrual period)
- 50–90 years of age
- Self-reported proficiency in speaking and understanding spoken English questions
- ≥8 years education
- Capable of cooperating for the duration of the study procedures and assessments
- Willing to undergo study procedures and remain unaware of the results (unless there are findings that are of clinical significance and would require further action, in the opinion of the study physician)

- Sufficient vision to participate in cognitive testing (corrected near visual acuity of Snellen 20/70 in at least one eye) and eye-tracking (able to identify symbols and stimuli presented on a computer screen in front of them)
- Sufficient corrected hearing to participate in cognitive testing
- Good venous access for phlebotomy to be performed
- Able to walk, with or without an assistive aid (e.g., cane, walker)

Subgroup-Specific Inclusion Criteria

Cognitively Normal Controls

- Cognitively normal and functionally independent in pre-screening history
- Within normal limits on the TorCA (formally known as Behavioural Neurology Assessment-Revised) (BNA-R)
- Within normal limits on the study neuropsychological battery

Mild Cognitive Impairment (MCI)

- Meets the National Institute on Aging-Alzheimer's Association criteria for single or multi-domain amnestic MCI
- Impairment of episodic memory plus or minus other cognitive domains on the TorCA
- Montreal Cognitive Assessment (MoCA) score ≥ 18
- Mini-Mental State Examination (MMSE) >20
- In the opinion of the investigator if required: a reliable and capable partner who has regular interaction with them, can provide a collateral history, can assist in compliance with study procedures, and who is willing to act as the Study Partner (provide written informed consent) and remain unaware of the results

Alzheimer's Disease (AD)

- Meets the National Institute on Aging-Alzheimer's Association (NIA-AA) core clinical criteria for probable or possible AD dementia
- Mild early AD stage, as defined by MMSE score ≥ 18, Atypical cases with a MoCA ≥ 14 will also be allowed
- Impairment in two or more cognitive domains on the TorCA
- Reliable and capable partner who has regular interaction with them, can provide a collateral history, can assist in compliance with study procedures, and who is willing to act as the Study Partner (provide written informed consent) and remain unaware of the results

Lewy Body Disease (LBD) Spectrum PD-MCI

- Meets the proposed Level I criteria for Mild Cognitive Impairment in Parkinson's Disease
- MMSE score ≥ 20
- MoCA score ≥ 18
- Impairment in one or more cognitive domains of TorCA

– Hoehn & Yahr stage 1–3
– Reliable and capable partner who has regular interaction with them, can provide a collateral history, can assist in compliance with study procedures, and who is willing to act as the Study Partner (provide written informed consent) and remain unaware of the results

LBD-MCI

– Meets the criteria for Dementia with Lewy Bodies but has preserved daily functioning
– MMSE score ≥ 20
– MoCA score ≥ 18
– Impairment in one or more cognitive domains on the TorCA
– Hoehn & Yahr stage ≤ 3
– Reliable and capable partner who has regular interaction with them, can provide a collateral history, can assist in compliance with study procedures, and who is willing to act as the Study Partner (provide written informed consent) and remain unaware of the results

Dementia with Lewy Bodies (DLB)

– Meets the criteria for probable or possible Dementia with Lewy Bodies
– MMSE score ≥ 14
– MoCA score ≤ 25
– Impairment in one or more cognitive domains on the TorCA
– Reliable and capable partner who has regular interaction with them, can provide a collateral history, can assist in compliance with study procedures, and who is willing to act as the Study Partner (provide written informed consent) and remain unaware of the results

PDD

– Meets the criteria for probable Parkinson's Disease—Dementia
– MMSE score ≥ 18
– MoCA score ≤ 25
– Impairment in two or more cognitive domains of TorCA
– Hoehn & Yahr stage ≤ 4
– Reliable and capable partner who has regular interaction with them, can provide a collateral history, can assist in compliance with study procedures, and who is willing to act as the Study Partner (provide written informed consent) and remain unaware of the results

Subcortical Vascular Cognitive Impairment (VCI)

• Presence of subcortical vascular disease, indicated by the following:
(a) Periventricular Fazekas score = 3, with or without subcortical lacunes or small cortical infarcts (<1.5 cm in longest diameter); or (b) Fazekas score ≥ 2, with 2 or more subcortical lacunes or small cortical infarcts (<1.5 cm in lon-

gest diameter); or (c) Fazekas score = 0 or 1, with 3 subcortical lacunar infarcts (<1.5 cm in diameter), at least 1 in each hemisphere; or (d) Probable or possible Cerebral Amyloid Angiopathy using the Modified Boston Criteria
- Impairment in one or more cognitive domains on the TorCA
- Reliable and capable partner who has regular interaction with them, can provide a collateral history, can assist in compliance with study procedures, and who is willing to act as the Study Partner (provide written informed consent) and remain unaware of the results

Exclusion Criteria General Exclusion Criteria (All Subgroups)

Participants who exhibit any of the following conditions will be excluded from the study:

- Underlying conditions (other than the disease being studied) which in the opinion of the investigator may interfere with the participant's ability to participate in the study or may compromise study results, including but not limited to:

  - Unstable cardiac, pulmonary, renal, hepatic, endocrine (i.e., diabetes) or hematologic disease
  - Active malignancy or infectious disease
  - Significant psychiatric illness, including life-long depressive illness
  - History of significant learning disability
  - Significant other neurologic disease (e.g., multiple sclerosis, Huntington's disease, normal pressure hydrocephalus, brain tumor, progressive supranuclear palsy, seizure disorder, subdural hematoma) or cognitive complications of cancer
  - Symptomatic stroke within the past 6 months
  - Substance abuse within the past year or history of alcohol or drug abuse which in the opinion of the investigator may interfere with the participant's ability to comply with the study procedures
  - History of significant head trauma or recurrent concussions requiring hospitalization followed by persistent neurologic defaults or known structural brain abnormalities
  - Pain or sleep disorder that could interfere with cognitive testing
  - Any disability that would limit the ability to perform study assessments

- Ocular conditions, including:
  (a) Clinical diagnosis of glaucoma, taking eye drops for glaucoma, or previous surgery (including laser) for glaucoma. (b) Any other serious eye disease or treatment or eye surgery, including any history of intra-vitreal injections. (c) History of optic neuritis. (d) Previous retinal laser therapy (either pan-retinal, or grid/focal) for diabetic retinopathy. (e) Cupping of the optic nerve head (ONH) is consistent with a diagnosis of glaucoma, as clinically determined by expert ophthalmological assessment of digital color fundus images centered on the ONH. Specifically, one or more of the following (assessed as part of SD-OCT visit at Kensington Eye Institute): (1) a cup/disc ratio of 0.7 or greater in either eye, (2) a cup/disc asymmetry of more than 0.2, (3) disc

hemorrhage, (4) notch, and (f) wet/exudative age-related macular degeneration (ARMD) in one or both eyes, as clinically determined by expert ophthalmological assessment of digital color fundus images centered on the fovea (assessed as part of SD-OCT visit at Kensington Eye Institute)

- Intra-ocular pressure greater than 22 mmHg or a difference in intra-ocular pressure (Goldmann tonometry) greater than 5 mmHg between the two eyes (assessed as part of SD-OCT visit at Kensington Eye Institute)
- Brain imaging abnormalities detected either on clinical MRI or CT prior to enrollment or on study MRI, including but not limited to:

  - Evidence of infection
  - Focal compressive mass lesions (tumors, subdural hematomas, malformations, etc.)

- Known hypersensitivity to Pittsburgh Compound B [11C]-PIB or any components of the [11C]-PIB Injection formulation
- Contraindications to 3 T MRI, as listed in the site-specific Magnetic Resonance Environment Screening Questionnaire (e.g., metal implant)
- Unable to tolerate the MRI environment (e.g., due to physical size and/or claustrophobia)
- Currently enrolled in a disease-modifying therapeutic trial that in the opinion of the Principal Investigator can potentially compromise study results

Subgroup-Specific Exclusion Criteria Cognitively Normal Controls

- Subjective memory complaints
- Brain imaging abnormalities detected either on clinical MRI or CT prior to enrollment or on study MRI, including but not limited to:

  - Periventricular Fazekas score = 2.5 or 3
  - Subcortical nonlacunar infarct or more than 1 subcortical lacunar infarct (<1.5 cm in longest diameter)
  - Cortical ischemic stroke Cortical or subcortical hemorrhagic stroke >1.5 cm in diameter

MCI, AD, and LBD Spectrum

- Brain imaging abnormalities detected either on clinical MRI or CT prior to enrollment or on study MRI, including but not limited to:

  - Periventricular Fazekas score = 2.5 or 3
  - Subcortical nonlacunar infarct or more than 1 subcortical lacunar infarct (<1.5 cm diameter)
  - Cortical ischemic stroke >1.5 cm in longest diameter
  - Cortical or subcortical hemorrhagic stroke >1.5 cm in diameter

Study Population

Three hundred and forty-five (345) participants will be enrolled: up to 85 cognitively normal elders, 65 with MCI, 65 with AD, 65 with LBD spectrum disease, and 65 with subcortical Vascular Cognitive Impairment.

All patients will receive a standardized work-up for dementia including brain imaging and a blood work screen to rule out secondary causes of dementia as part of their clinical work-up prior to study enrollment. Memory clinic patients will undergo a detailed neurocognitive assessment (Toronto Cognitive Assessment—TorCA), and the clinical history and examination will use a standardized common elements approach.

Ages Eligible for Study
50 Years to 90 Years (Adult, Older Adult)

Sexes Eligible for Study
All

Accepts Healthy Volunteers
Yes

Sampling Method
Non-Probability Sample

Observational Model: Cohort
Time Perspective: Cross-Sectional
Biospecimen Retention: Samples with DNA
Biospecimen Description: Blood samples for genetic testing including apolipoprotein E4 status, as well as for proteomic, lipidomic, and other fluid biomarkers of neurodegeneration and vascular disease, will be collected for each participant. All samples should be taken after a 10 h fast; if not possible, the participant should have a light meal only. Samples should be collected between 8 am and 10 am, in order to minimize circadian variations in biomarker levels.

Cohorts and interventions

Group/cohort	Intervention/treatment
Normal controls Up to 85 normal elders, 50–90 years old who are within normal limits on the study neuropsychological battery will be enrolled. All patients involved in the study will undergo SD-OCT, eye tracking, gait and balance assessments, blood draw for genomics and fluid biomarkers, neuropsychological assessment, brain MRI, and brain amyloid PET	Other: Pittsburgh Compound B [11C]-PIB • This is a cross-sectional study of patients with various forms of cognitive impairment and a healthy control group for comparison. Brain amyloid PET scans using the radioligand Pittsburgh Compound B [11C]-PIB, which is not yet approved for clinical use in Canada, will be performed in all subjects

Group/cohort	Intervention/treatment
Alzheimer's disease (AD) Sixty-five subjects meeting the National Institute on Aging-Alzheimer's Association (NIA-AA) core clinical criteria for probable AD dementia will be enrolled. All patients will undergo SD-OCT, eye tracking, gait and balance assessments, blood draw for genomics and fluid biomarkers, neuropsychological assessment, brain MRI, and brain amyloid PET. A subset will undergo SV-OCT	Other: Pittsburgh Compound B [11C]-PIB • This is a cross-sectional study of patients with various forms of cognitive impairment and a healthy control group for comparison. Brain amyloid PET scans using the radioligand Pittsburgh Compound B [11C]-PIB, which is not yet approved for clinical use in Canada, will be performed in all subjects
Mild Cognitive Impairment (VCI) Sixty-five subjects meeting the National Institute on Aging-Alzheimer's Association criteria for amnestic or multi-domain MCI with MoCA score ≥ 18 will be enrolled. All patients will undergo SD-OCT, eye tracking, gait and balance assessments, blood draw for genomics and fluid biomarkers, neuropsychological assessment, brain MRI and brain amyloid PET. A subset will undergo SV-OCT	Other: Pittsburgh Compound B [11C]-PIB • This is a cross-sectional study of patients with various forms of cognitive impairment and a healthy control group for comparison. Brain amyloid PET scans using the radioligand Pittsburgh Compound B [11C]-PIB, which is not yet approved for clinical use in Canada, will be performed in all subjects
Subcortical Vascular Impairment (VCI) Sixty-five subjects meeting the American Heart Association-American Stroke Association (AHA-ASA) criteria for probable vascular dementia (VaD) or probable vascular mild cognitive impairment (VaMCI) due to subcortical ischemic vascular disease, and probable or possible Cerebral Amyloid Angiopathy using the Modified Boston Criteria will be enrolled. All patients will undergo SD-OCT, eye tracking, gait and balance assessments, blood draw for genomics and fluid biomarkers, neuropsychological assessment, brain MRI, and brain amyloid PET. A subset will undergo SV-OCT	Other: Pittsburgh Compound B [11C]-PIB • This is a cross-sectional study of patients with various forms of cognitive impairment and a healthy control group for comparison. Brain amyloid PET scans using the radioligand Pittsburgh Compound B [11C]-PIB, which is not yet approved for clinical use in Canada, will be performed in all subjects
LBD Spectrum Sixty-five subjects with Dementia with Lewy Bodies (DLB) meeting the criteria for probable Dementia with Lewy Bodies with MMSE score ≥ 20; or PD-MCI meeting the proposed Level I criteria for Mild Cognitive Impairment in Parkinson's Disease with MoCA score 18–24; or; PDD meeting the criteria for probable Parkinson's Disease—Dementia and MMSE score ≥ 20 will be enrolled. All patients involved will undergo SD-OCT, eye tracking, gait and balance assessments, blood draw for genomics and fluid biomarkers, neuropsychological assessment, brain MRI and brain amyloid PET. A subset will undergo SV-OCT	Other: Pittsburgh Compound B [11C]-PIB • This is a cross-sectional study of patients with various forms of cognitive impairment and a healthy control group for comparison. Brain amyloid PET scans using the radioligand Pittsburgh Compound B [11C]-PIB, which is not yet approved for clinical use in Canada, will be performed in all subjects

Primary outcome measures

Outcome measure	Measure description	Time frame
Retinal nerve fiber layer thickness	This potential ocular biomarker will be compared among the different cohorts and be validated against brain MRI and brain amyloid PET	One-time assessment
Amyloid deposition	This will be compared among the different cohorts and be validated against brain amyloid PET, and are expected to correlate meaningfully with cognitive and behavioral patterns, including retinal and eye-tracking, gait and balance	One-time assessment

Secondary outcome measures

Outcome measure	Measure description	Time frame
Retinal artery narrowing	The extent of the correlation between retinal artery narrowing and the presence of covert lacunar infarcts on MRI will be assessed	One-time assessment
Retinal venular widening	The extent of the correlation between retinal venular widening and the amount of periventricular white matter hyperintensities on MRI will be assessed	One-time assessment

Sponsor
Sunnybrook Health Sciences Centre

Collaborators
- Brain Canada
- Weston Brain Institute
- GE Healthcare
- University Health Network, Toronto
- Centre for Addiction and Mental Health
- Baycrest
- Unity Health Toronto
- Kensington Eye Institute

Investigators
- Principal Investigator: Sandra Black, MD, Sunnybrook Health Sciences Center

General Publications

No publications available

Light Intervention

Recruiting

United States

Light, Metabolic Syndrome and Alzheimer's Disease: Aim 2

ClinicalTrials.gov ID NCT03933696

Sponsor Icahn School of Medicine at Mount Sinai
Information provided by Mariana Figueiro, Icahn School of Medicine at Mount Sinai (Responsible Party)
Last Update Posted 2023-09-13

Brief Summary
To test the long-term effect of light treatment on cognition, sleep, and metabolism in patients with mild cognitive impairment (MCI) or mild Alzheimer's disease or related dementia (ADRD).

Detailed Description
Test if a tailored light intervention (TLI) that promotes entrainment can improve sleep disturbances, inflammation, insulin sensitivity (Si), glucose disposal (Sg), and cognition in patients with MCI and mild ADRD and sleep disturbances. Using a single-arm, between-subjects, placebo-controlled study the investigators will investigate if long-term (6-month) exposure to TLI improves glucose homeostasis and insulin sensitivity in patients with MCI and mild AD who suffer from sleep disturbance and are living at home. Participants will be recruited from the Mount Sinai AD research center (ADRC) and randomized to receive the TLI (or comparison control treatment) at home. The investigators hypothesize that, compared to the comparison light, a TLI will increase entrainment, improve sleep, reduce depression, reduce inflammation, improve metabolic control, increase insulin sensitivity, and reduce susceptibility to T2DM and metabolic disease during and after the completion of the 6-month intervention.

Official Title
Light, Metabolic Syndrome and Alzheimer's Disease: A Non-Pharmacological Approach

Conditions
Mild Cognitive Impairment
Alzheimer Disease
Type 2 Diabetes

Intervention/Treatment
- Device: Tailored Lighting Intervention

Other Study ID Numbers
- GCO 17-2685-0002

Study Start (Actual)
2019-01-02

Primary Completion (Estimated)
2024-05-31

Study Completion (Estimated)
2024-05-31

Enrollment (Estimated)
30

Study Type
Interventional

Phase
Not Applicable

Study Contact
Name: Christoph Buettner, MD, PhD
Phone Number: 212-241-3425
Email: cb1116@rwjms.rutgers.edu

Study Contact Backup
Name: Barbara Plitnick, RN
Phone Number: 518-242-4603
Email: barbara.plitnick@mountsinai.org
United States
New Jersey Locations

New Brunswick, New Jersey, United States, 08854
Recruiting
Rutgers University

Contact
Christoph Buettner, MD
cb1116@rwjms.rutgers.edu

New York Locations

New York, New York, United States, 10029
Recruiting
Icahn School of Medicine at Mount Sinai

Contact
Christoph Buettner, MD, PhD
212-241-3425 christoph.buettner@mssm.edu

Inclusion Criteria
- Mild cognitive impairment
- Mild Alzheimer's Disease
- Sleep Disturbance
- Live at home

Exclusion Criteria
- Blindness
- insulin-dependent diabetes patients
- macular degeneration
- severe sleep apnea

Ages Eligible for Study
55 Years and older (Adult, Older Adult)

Sexes Eligible for Study
All

Accepts Healthy Volunteers
No

Design Details
Primary Purpose: Treatment
Allocation: Randomized
Interventional Model: Parallel Assignment
Interventional Model Description: Participants will be randomly assigned to receive the active or placebo lighting condition
Masking: Double (Participant Care Provider)

Arms and interventions

Participant group/arm	Intervention/treatment
Active comparator: active lighting intervention The TLI will provide high circadian stimulation during the day produced by light sources that provide moderate light levels of spectra that are tuned to the sensitivity of the circadian system. Combining spectrum and light level, TLI will allow us to (a) use a light source that will stimulate the circadian system and (b) provide the participants with options as to how the light treatment will be delivered. The investigators will deliver at least 300–400 lux at the eye of the bluish-white light during the day (CS of 0.4 or greater) The lighting intervention will be in place for 24 weeks	Device: tailored lighting intervention • Lighting intervention either active or placebo
Placebo comparator: placebo lighting intervention The placebo condition light source will be a warm yellow-white (2700–3000 K) source providing 50–100 lux at the eye. The lighting intervention will be in place for 24 weeks	Device: tailored lighting intervention • Lighting intervention either active or placebo

Primary outcome measures

Outcome measure	Measure description	Time frame
Sleep disturbance	Change in sleep disturbance will be assessed using the Pittsburgh Sleep Quality Index. The sum of the 7 component scores yields a single global score. A person with a global score above 5 is considered to have sleep disturbances. A higher score indicates worsening sleep disturbance	Done at baseline, week 13, 25 and 48
Metabolic control	Changes in glucose homeostasis and insulin sensitivity will be measured using the Frequently Sampled Intravenous Glucose Tolerance Test (FSIVGTT)	Done at baseline, week 13 and 25
Depression	A change in depression will be assessed using the Cornell Scale for Depression in Dementia. A score of 9 or more points indicates depression	Done at baseline, week 13, 25 and 48
Cognition	Changes in cognition will be assessed by the use of the Alzheimer's Disease Assessment Scale-Cognitive Sub scale (ADAS-Cog). All scores are summed and higher scores indicate a higher severity of dementia	Done at baseline, week 13, 25 and 48
Cognition	Changes in cognition will be assessed using the mini mental state exam (MMSE). All scores are summed for a total score ranging from 0 to 30. A lower score indicates worsening dementia	Done at baseline, week 13, 25 and 48

Secondary outcome measures

Outcome measure	Measure description	Time frame
Sleep disturbance using actigraphy	Actigraphs will be worn for 7 days during assessment weeks to measure sleep	Done at baseline, week 13, 25 and 48
Light measurements	Light measurements will be collected using the Daysimeter for 7 days	Done at baseline, week 13, 25 and 48
Melatonin levels	First morning urine will be collected and assayed for melatonin levels	One morning during baseline, week 13, 25, and 48

Sponsor
Icahn School of Medicine at Mount Sinai

Investigators
- Principal Investigator: Mariana G Figueiro, PhD, Icahn School of Medicine at Mount Sinai

General Publications

No publications available

Retina

Recruiting

Austria

Retinal Neuro-Vascular Coupling in Patients with Neurodegenerative Disease

ClinicalTrials.gov ID NCT02663531

Sponsor Medical University of Vienna
Information provided by Gerhard Garhofer, Medical University of Vienna
    (Responsible Party)
Last Update Posted 2022-04-07

Brief Summary
Alzheimer's disease (AD) is one of the most important causes of dementia and poses a considerable challenge in health care. Today, criteria for the diagnosis and the follow-up of patients with AD mainly rely either on subjective tests or invasive methods. This limits the general applicability of the latter test for population screening and underlines the need for the identification of easily accessible tools for the identification of high-risk subjects. Because of its unique optical properties, the eye offers the possibility of the noninvasive assessment of both structural and functional alterations in neuronal tissue. As the neuro-retina is part of the brain, it does not come as a surprise that neuro-degenerative changes in the brain are accompanied by structural and possibly also functional changes in the neuro-retina and the ocular vasculature.

The current study seeks to test the hypothesis that besides the known anatomical changes, also functional changes can be detected in the retina of patients with AD. For this purpose, flicker light-induced hyperemia will be measured in the retina as a functional test to assess the coupling between neural activity and blood flow. Furthermore, structural parameters such as retinal nerve fiber layer thickness and function parameters such as ocular blood flow and retinal oxygenation will be assessed and compared to age- and sex-matched controls.

Official Title
Retinal Neuro-vascular Coupling in Patients with Neurodegenerative Disease

Conditions
Mild Cognitive Impairment
Alzheimer Disease
Healthy

Intervention/Treatment
- Device: DVA
- Device: FDOCT
- Device: Pattern ERG
- Device: Optical Coherence Tomography

Other Study ID Numbers

- OPHT-180515

Study Start (Actual)

2016-09-27

Primary Completion (Estimated)

2023-09

Study Completion (Estimated)

2023-09-30

Enrollment (Estimated)

150

Study Type

Interventional

Phase

Not Applicable

Study Contact

Name: Gerhard Garhöfer, MD
Phone Number: 0043140400 ext 29810
Email: gerhard.garhoefer@medunwien.ac.at
Austria

Vienna, Austria, 1090
Recruiting
Department of Clinical Pharmacology, Medical University of Vienna

Contact

Gerhard Garhöfer, MD
+43 (1) 40400 ext 29810 gerhard.garhoefer@meduniwien.ac.at

Principal Investigator

Gerhard Garhöfer, MD

Inclusion Criteria

Inclusion criteria for healthy subjects:

- Men and women aged over 50 years
- Nonsmokers
- Normal findings in the medical history unless the investigator considers an abnormality to be clinically irrelevant
- Normal ophthalmic findings, ametropia <6 Dpt

Inclusion criteria for patients with AD:

- Men and women aged over 50 years
- Normal ophthalmic findings, ametropia <6 Dpt
- Confirmed diagnosis of probable AD of mild to moderate degree defined as:

- Diagnosis of probable Alzheimer's disease based on the NINCDS/ADRDA criteria
- Assessing the severity of Alzheimer's disease of mild to moderate degree by the Mini Mental State Examination (MMSE). AD of mild to moderate degree has been confirmed if the MMSE score is in the range of 20–26 inclusive

- The Hachinski Ischemia Scale is used to try and distinguish AD from multi-infarct dementia. A score of ≤ 4 suggests AD Informed consent capability
- Adequate visual and auditory acuity to allow neuropsychological testing and participation in the ocular blood flow measurements
- A potential participant has to be on stable doses of all medications he/she is taking because of consistent illnesses according to medical history (except AD therapy, which will be recorded separately) for at least 30 days prior to inclusion, if considered relevant by the investigator.

Inclusion criteria for patients with mild cognitive impairment:

- Men and women aged over 50 years
- Normal ophthalmic findings, ametropia <6 Dpt.
- Diagnosis of probable mild cognitive impairment (MCI) defined as:

  - Memory complaint, corroborated by an informant
  - Abnormal memory function, documented by the delayed recall of one paragraph from the Logical Memory II subtest of the Wechsler Memory Scale-Revised (cutoff scores: ≤ 8 for ≥ 16 years of education; ≤ 4 for 8–15 years of education; and ≤ 2 for 0–7 years of education [the maximum number of paragraph items possible to correctly recall is 25])
  - Normal general cognitive function, as determined by a clinician's judgment based on a structured interview with the patient and an informant (Clinical Dementia Rating [CDR]) and a Mini-Mental State Examination (MMSE) score greater than 26
  - No or minimal impairment in activities of daily living (ADLs), as determined by a clinical interview with the patient and informant
  - Not sufficiently impaired, cognitively and functionally, to meet the NINCDS/ADRDA criteria, as judged by an experienced AD research clinician

- The Hachinski Ischemia Scale is used to try and distinguish MCI from multi-infarct dementia. A score of ≤ 4 suggests MCI Informed consent capability
- Adequate visual and auditory acuity to allow neuropsychological testing and participation in the ocular blood flow measurements
- A potential participant has to be on stable doses of all medications he/she is taking because of consistent illnesses according to medical for at least 30 days prior to inclusion, if considered relevant by the investigator.

Exclusion Criteria for patients:

- Presence or history of a severe medical condition other than cognitive impairment as judged by the clinical investigator
- Untreated Arterial hypertension
- History or family history of epilepsy
- Presence of any abnormalities preventing reliable measurements in the study eye as judged by the investigator
- Best corrected visual acuity <0.5 Snellen
- Ametropia greater than 6 Dpt
- Pregnancy or planned pregnancy
- Major psychiatric disorder (e.g., schizophrenia), if considered relevant by the investigator
- Significant neurological disease other than AD or MCI, if considered relevant by the investigator
- Alcoholism or substance abuse

Exclusion criteria for healthy volunteers:

- Presence or history of a severe medical condition as judged by the clinical investigator
- Untreated Arterial hypertension
- History or family history of epilepsy
- Presence of any abnormalities preventing reliable measurements in the study eye as judged by the investigator
- Family history of AD
- Best corrected visual acuity <0.5 Snellen
- Ametropia 6 Dpt
- Pregnancy or planned pregnancy

Ages Eligible for Study
50 Years and older (Adult, Older Adult)

Sexes Eligible for Study
All

Accepts Healthy Volunteers
Yes

Primary Purpose: Basic Science
Allocation: Randomized
Interventional Model: Parallel Assignment
Masking: None (Open Label)

Arms and interventions

Participant group/arm	Intervention/treatment
Experimental: mild cognitive impairment Patients with mild cognitive impairment	Device: DVA • Other names: – Dynamic Vessel Analyzer Device: FDOCT • Other names: – Fourier Domain Color Doppler Optical Coherence Tomography Device: Pattern ERG Device: Optical Coherence Tomography
Experimental: Alzheimer's Disease Patients with Alzheimer's Disease	Device: DVA • Other names: – Dynamic Vessel Analyzer Device: FDOCT • Other names: – Fourier Domain Color Doppler Optical Coherence Tomography Device: Paturation for participantstern ERG Device: Optical Coherence Tomography
Experimental: Healthy Healthy volunteers	Device: DVA • Other names: – Dynamic Vessel Analyzer Device: FDOCT • Other names: – Fourier Domain Color Doppler Optical Coherence Tomography Device: Pattern ERG Device: Optical Coherence Tomography

Primary outcome measures

Outcome measure	Measure description	Time frame
Flicker-induced increase in retinal blood flow		1 day

Sponsor
Medical University of Vienna

Collaborators
No information provided

Investigators
• Principal Investigator: Gerhard Garhöfer, MD, Department of Clinical Pharmacology, Medical University of Vienna

General Publications

No publications available

Retina

Recruiting

Belgium

Multimodal Retinal Imaging in the Detection and Follow-Up of Alzheimer's Disease (RetAD)

ClinicalTrials.gov ID NCT03466177

Sponsor Universitaire Ziekenhuizen KU Leuven
Information provided by Universitaire Ziekenhuizen KU Leuven (Responsible Party)
Last Update Posted 2023-10-10

Brief Summary

Because of a shared ontogenic origin, the retina displays similarities to the brain and spinal cord in terms of anatomy, functionality, response to insult, and immunology. Hence, the retina can be approached as an integral part of the central nervous system. The occurrence of ocular manifestations in several neurodegenerative pathologies, such as Alzheimer's disease and Parkinson's disease, accentuates the strong relationship between the eye and brain. Particularly retinal changes can present a substrate for cerebral changes in these disorders. Offering a 'window to the brain', the transparent eye enables non-invasive imaging of these changes in retinal structure and vasculature. In this project, the potential of retinal biomarkers for, e.g., Alzheimer's will be explored with the aim to overcome some of the hurdles in the current management of these pathologies, mainly the lack of techniques for patient screening and early diagnosis. The aim of this clinical trial is to correlate the retinal biomarkers for Alzheimer's with neuro-imaging and cognitive function. Integrating the results will yield noninvasive retinal biomarkers for clinical research, screening, and follow-up of disease progression in various neurodegenerative disorders.

Detailed Description

Alzheimer's disease (AD) is the most common neurodegenerative disorder and the leading cause of dementia worldwide. A growing number of people are surviving into their 80s–90s and the number of AD patients is projected to nearly triple in the next three decades, affecting 80–90 million people worldwide by 2040. As such, AD will become the third cause of death for older people, just behind cardiovascular disease and cancer. In contrast to the latter, AD cannot be prevented, slowed, or cured. AD represents an enormous socio-economic burden and has become a trillion dollar disease. Despite decades of intensive research, diagnosis and treatment remain challenging for AD. A string of recent failures in clinical trials for AD drugs has pointed out that our understanding of the disease is still far from complete. More in detail, three major reasons underlying this treatment gap have been identified:

1. The lack of techniques for patient screening and early diagnosis

2. The incomplete understanding of the complex interplay of pathological processes that underlie AD
3. The many hurdles between drug discovery and approval

With this study, the investigators propose a novel way to address these needs, by using the retina as a model organ to study the central nervous system (CNS). Many of the hallmark cerebral pathophysiological processes of AD have also been observed in the retina. Unlike the rest of the CNS, the retina can be visualized directly, with an imaging resolution up to 100× higher than PET and MRI scans. Using these high-resolution imaging tools such as Optical Coherence Tomography (OCT), studies have demonstrated microvascular changes and neuro-retinal thinning in AD patients. Pilot data show that retinal Aβ can be visualized noninvasively solely based on the intrinsic hyperspectral signature of aggregated amyloid deposits. Noninvasive retinal imaging (e.g., fundus photography, OCT, hyperspectral imaging (HSI))—which are all available at affordable cost—, could therefore represent novel means for identifying patients at risk, for longitudinal follow-up of disease progression in AD patients, and for research in a quest for more effective treatments.

This is an open-label longitudinal biomarker study without investigational medicinal product in subjects in different stages of the AD spectrum.

The data that we will collect consist of amyloid imaging, MRI, blood, genetic, general health, and cognitive data, as well as visual acuity, ocular biomicroscopy and funduscopy, fundus photographs, hyperspectral retinal images, Optical Coherence Tomography (OCT) retinal images, and OCT angiography (OCT-A) retinal images. Subjects will be followed longitudinally. In the current study, the investigators will primarily investigate the potential of noninvasive, multimodal retinal imaging for the early detection of Alzheimer's disease and for the evaluation of disease progression. This will be done in comparison with amyloid imaging and neuropsychological evaluations.

The investigators will build a longitudinal database of ocular, systemic, neuropsychiatric, MRI, and PET imaging parameters of Aβ-positive and Aβ-negative patients with different stages of cognitive impairment. This database will be used to provide proof-of-concept that retinal biomarkers provide an early, accurate, and non-invasive tool for AD detection and follow-up. All data will be collected in a database for statistical analysis.

Official Title
Multimodal Retinal Imaging in the Detection and Follow-up of Alzheimer's Disease

Conditions
Alzheimer Disease
Alzheimer Dementia
Mild Cognitive Impairment
Dementia
Glaucoma
Age-Related Macular Degeneration
Diabetic Retinopathy

Intervention/Treatment
- Diagnostic Test: Noninvasive, multimodal retinal imaging

Other Study ID Numbers
- S60932

Study Start (Actual)
2018-03-01

Primary Completion (Estimated)
2024-12-31

Study Completion (Estimated)
2025-12-31

Enrollment (Estimated)
320

Study Type
Observational

Study Contact
Name: Jan Van Eijgen, MD
Phone Number: +3216332387
Email: jan.1.vaneijgen@uzleuven.be
Belgium
Vlaams Brabant Locations

Leuven, Vlaams Brabant, Belgium, 3000
Recruiting
UZ Leuven

Contact
Ingeborg Stalmans, Phd
003216332372 ingeborg.stalmans@uzleuven.be

Contact
Sarah Spileers, Optometrist
003216340391 oogziekten.glaucoomstudies@uzleuven.be

Sub-Investigator
Rik Vandenberghe, MD, PHD

Inclusion Criteria
- Between ≥50 and ≤85 years of age
- In the opinion of the investigator, the patient is in stable medical condition and willing and able to perform study procedures
- Patient is fluent in written and verbal Dutch
- Patient is capable of giving informed consent

Exclusion Criteria

- Patient has a history or current evidence of a neurological disorder, which, in the opinion of the primary investigator, may contribute to the subject's cognitive impairment.
- Patient has a history of large-vessel stroke or evidence of a large-vessel infarction or other focal lesions on baseline MRI scan, which may contribute to the cause of the memory impairment in the opinion of the investigator. Vascular white matter lesions or other signs of microangiopathy will not be considered an exclusion.
- Patient has a history of malignancy $\leq$5 years prior to signing informed consent, except for patients who have undergone potentially curative therapy with no evidence of recurrence for 1 year, and who are deemed at low risk for recurrency by her/his treating physician.
- Patient is currently participating or has participated in a study with an investigational compound within 30 days of signing informed consent.
- Subject has any magnetizable metal prostheses, implants, or foreign objects that could pose a hazard during MRI scans.
- Patient has a known history of ocular diseases other than the exception of cataract and/or wearing glasses/contact lenses.

Study Population
Cfr. eligibility criteria

Ages Eligible for Study
50 Years to 85 Years (Adult, Older Adult)

Sexes Eligible for Study
All

Sampling Method
Probability Sample

Observational Model: Cohort
Time Perspective: Prospective

Cohorts and interventions

Group/cohort	Intervention/treatment
Ab+ AD patients Amyloid positive Alzheimer's disease patients – Ocular examination visual acuity, biomicroscopy, funduscopy fundus pictures, including hyperspectral imaging OCT + angio-OCT (non-invasive, multimodal retinal imaging), Dynamic Vessel Analyzer (DVA)	Diagnostic test: noninvasive, multimodal retinal imaging • Ocular exam including the application of different noninvasive ocular imaging techniques
Ab+ mild cognitive impairment (MCI) patients Amyloid positive mild cognitive impairment patients – Ocular examination visual acuity, biomicroscopy, funduscopy fundus pictures, including hyperspectral imaging OCT + angio-OCT (non-invasive, multimodal retinal imaging), Dynamic Vessel Analyzer (DVA)	Diagnostic test: noninvasive, multimodal retinal imaging • Ocular exam including the application of different noninvasive ocular imaging techniques

Group/cohort	Intervention/treatment
Ab+ cognitively intact volunteers Amyloid positive cognitively intact volunteers – Ocular examination visual acuity, biomicroscopy, funduscopy fundus pictures, including hyperspectral imaging OCT + angio-OCT (noninvasive, multimodal retinal imaging), Dynamic Vessel Analyzer (DVA)	Diagnostic test: noninvasive, multimodal retinal imaging • Ocular exam including the application of different noninvasive ocular imaging techniques
Ab−cognitively intact volunteers Amyloid negative cognitively intact volunteers – Ocular examination visual acuity, biomicroscopy, funduscopy, fundus pictures, including hyperspectral imaging OCT + angio-OCT (non-invasive, multimodal retinal imaging), and Dynamic Vessel Analyzer (DVA)	Diagnostic test: noninvasive, multimodal retinal imaging • Ocular exam including the application of different noninvasive ocular imaging techniques
Glaucoma patients –Ocular examination visual acuity, biomicroscopy, funduscopy, fundus pictures, including hyperspectral imaging OCT + angio-OCT (noninvasive, multimodal retinal imaging), and Dynamic Vessel Analyzer (DVA)	Diagnostic test: noninvasive, multimodal retinal imaging • Ocular exam including the application of different noninvasive ocular imaging techniques
Age-related macular degeneration patients – Ocular examination visual acuity, biomicroscopy, funduscopy, fundus pictures, including hyperspectral imaging OCT + angio-OCT (noninvasive, multimodal retinal imaging), and Dynamic Vessel Analyzer (DVA)	Diagnostic test: noninvasive, multimodal retinal imaging • Ocular exam including the application of different noninvasive ocular imaging techniques
Diabetic retinopathy patients – Ocular examination visual acuity, biomicroscopy, funduscopy, fundus pictures, including hyperspectral imaging OCT + angio-OCT (non-invasive, multimodal retinal imaging), and DVA	Diagnostic test: noninvasive, multimodal retinal imaging • Ocular exam including the application of different noninvasive ocular imaging techniques

Primary outcome measures

Outcome measure	Measure description	Time frame
Retinal biomarkers for AD: specificity	To evaluate the diagnostic performance of selected ocular biomarkers for Alzheimer's disease	5 years
Retinal biomarkers for AD: sensitivity	To evaluate the diagnostic performance of selected ocular biomarkers for Alzheimer's disease	5 years
Retinal biomarkers for AD: number needed to image	To evaluate the diagnostic performance of selected ocular biomarkers for Alzheimer's disease	5 years
Retinal biomarkers for AD: area under the curve (AUC)	To evaluate the diagnostic performance of selected ocular biomarkers for Alzheimer's disease	5 years
Retinal biomarkers for AD: receiver operating characteristic (ROC)	To evaluate the diagnostic performance of selected ocular biomarkers for Alzheimer's disease	5 years

Secondary outcome measures

Outcome measure	Measure description	Time frame
Retinal biomarkers for AD: quantification of cerebral Aβ load by noninvasive retinal imaging against the cerebral Aβ load measured by cerebral imaging	To deliver a proof-of-concept for the use of retinal biomarkers to quantitatively measure cerebral Aβ load by comparing the results of cerebral imaging (Standard Uptake Value ratio (SUVr) on amyloid-PET) with the results of retinal hyperspectral imaging (area of retinal Aβ detected, in μm²)	15 years
Retinal biomarkers for AD: disease progression by measuring the change from baseline at 2 years and more	To deliver a proof-of-concept for the use of retinal biomarkers to follow Alzheimer's disease progression by measuring the change from baseline at 2 years and after and to compare the results of the cerebral imaging and neuropsychiatric tests with the results from the selected retinal biomarkers for AD at different time points (t0, t 6 months, t 12 months, t 18 months, t 24 months, yearly for 15 years)	15 years

Sponsor
Universitaire Ziekenhuizen KU Leuven

Collaborators
No information provided

Investigators
- Principal Investigator: Ingeborg Stalmans, MD, PhD, UZ Leuven/KU Leuven

General Publications

No publications available

Retina

Recruiting

France

Finding Retinal Biomarkers in Alzheimer's Disease (FIREBALZ)

ClinicalTrials.gov ID NCT05067010

Sponsor Assistance Publique - Hôpitaux de Paris
Information provided by Assistance Publique—Hôpitaux de Paris (Responsible Party)
Last Update Posted 2023-03-06

Brief Summary

CSF Alzheimer's disease (AD) biomarkers are the one that reflects both Aβ and tau pathologies. There is increasing evidence for the presence of AD abnormalities in the retina of AD patients. Recent studies showed that they can be detected in living patients. Thus, retinal AD-linked abnormalities might be used as alternative diagnostic biomarkers for AD.

FIREBALZ study aims to identify and validate retinal biomarkers for diagnosing of Alzheimer's disease.

The study will include 160 patients in whom LP is indicated for the assessment of CSF AD biomarkers according to French Health Authority (HAS) recommendations. Those patients will undergo a detailed neuro-ophthalmologic evaluation including retinal layers thickness evaluation (optical coherence tomography).

Univariate and multivariate analyses will be performed to test diagnostic properties of retinal parameters as compared to current diagnostic criteria including CSF biomarkers and logistic regression models will be used.

Detailed Description

Cerebrospinal fluid (CSF) Alzheimer's disease (AD) biomarkers are the one that reflects both Aβ and tau pathologies. There is increasing evidence for the presence of AD abnormalities in the retina of AD patients. Recent studies showed that they can be detected in living patients. Thus, retinal AD-linked abnormalities might be used as alternative diagnostic biomarkers for AD.

FIREBALZ study aims to identify and validate retinal biomarkers for diagnosing of Alzheimer's disease.

The study will include 160 patients in whom lumbar puncture is indicated for the assessment of CSF AD biomarkers according to French health authority recommendations. All patients will be recruited at the Cognitive Neurology Center (CMRR Paris Nord Ile-De-France), Paris, France. Patients will undergo a detailed neuro-ophthalmologic evaluation including a complete ophthalmologic work-up to rule out chronic retinal pathology and retinal layers thickness evaluation (optical coherence tomography).

The inclusion period will be 40.5 months, Study duration for participants will be 6–12 weeks.

Two groups of patients will be defined for comparison according to LP results: patients with AD according to McKhann criteria and patients without AD Univariate and multivariate analyses will be performed to test diagnostic properties of retinal parameters and logistic regression models will be used.

Official Title

Finding Retinal Biomarkers in Alzheimer's Disease

Conditions

Alzheimer Disease

Intervention/Treatment

- Other: Detailed ophthalmologic examination

Other Study ID Numbers
- D20170821

Study Start (Actual)
2021-06-10

Primary Completion (Actual)
2021-09-30

Study Completion (Estimated)
2024-12-24

Enrollment (Estimated)
160

Study Type
Observational [Patient Registry]

Study Contact
Name: Emmanuel COGNAT, Dr.
Phone Number: 01 40 05 49 54
Email: emmanuel.cognat@aphp.fr
France

Paris, France, 75010
Recruiting
Centre Mémoire de Ressources et de Recherche Paris Nord

Contact
Claire PAQUET, MD, PhD
33 6 84 18 28 34 claire.paquet@inserm.fr

Eligibility Criteria
Description

Inclusion Criteria
- Patient managed at the cognitive neurology center for cognitive impairment with a defined LP indication for the assessment of CSF AD biomarkers according to French National Health Agency recommendations in a clinical practice setting
- Patients with National Health Insurance coverage
- Patients willing to participate in the research and sign informed consent

Exclusion Criteria
- Patient refusing to participate in research or unable to sign an informed consent
- Patients without indication or displaying contraindication of LP
- Chronic retinal pathology interfering with analysis:

  - Chronic glaucoma
  - Diabetic retinopathy
  - Severe hypertensive retinopathy

- Contraindication to brain MRI
- Other pathology considered as severe and impairing life expectancy

Study Population

Patients in whom lumbar puncture (LP) is indicated for assessment of CSF AD biomarkers according to French health authority (HAS) recommendations. All patients will be recruited at the Cognitive Neurology Center (CMRR Paris Nord Ile-De-France), Paris, France. Patients will undergo a detailed neuro-ophthalmologic evaluation including a complete ophthalmologic work-up to rule out chronic retinal pathology and retinal layers thickness evaluation (optical coherence tomography).

The inclusion period will be 40.5 months, Study duration for participants will be 6 to 12 weeks.

Two groups of patients will be defined for comparison according to LP results: patients with AD (MCI and Dementia) according to McKhann criteria and patients without AD Univariate and multivariate analyses will be performed to test diagnostic properties of retinal parameters and logistic regression models will be used.

Ages Eligible for Study
(Child, Adult, Older Adult)

Sexes Eligible for Study
All

Accepts Healthy Volunteers
No

Sampling Method
Probability Sample

Design Details
Observational Model: Cohort
Time Perspective: Prospective
Target Follow-up Duration: 52 Months

Cohorts and interventions

Intervention/treatment

Other: detailed ophthalmologic examination
  • Visual acuity
  • Eye pressure measurement
  • Eye crystalline examination
  • Fundus examination
  • Optical coherence tomography of the retina
  • Retinal photos

Primary outcome measures

Outcome measure	Measure description	Time frame
Diagnostic properties of retinal layer thickness measurement using OCT	Diagnostic properties of retinal layers thickness measurement using OCT for the diagnosis of probable AD according to McKhann criteria combining clinical criteria and CSF biomarker results	Up to 6 at 12 weeks

Secondary outcome measures

Outcome measure	Measure description	Time frame
The diagnostic properties of optical coherence tomography (OCT) and retinal photos for the diagnosis of Alzheimer's disease	The diagnostic properties of optical coherence tomography (OCT) and retinal photos for the diagnosis of Alzheimer's disease	Up to 6 at 12 weeks
Relationship between retinal layer thickness measurements and retinal abnormalities	Relationship between retinal layer thickness measurements and retinal abnormalities	Up to 6 at 12 weeks
Relationship between retinal layer thickness measurements and markers of clinical	Relationship between retinal layer thickness measurements and markers of clinical	Up to 6 at 12 weeks
Relationship between retinal layer thickness measurements and imaging severity	Relationship between retinal layer thickness measurements and imaging (hippocampal volume and cortical atrophy evaluated semi-quantitatively on brain MRI) severity	Up to 6 at 12 weeks
The diagnostic properties of optical coherence tomography (OCT) and retinal photos for the diagnosis of cognitive alteration of neurodegenerative origin (all causes)	The diagnostic properties of optical coherence tomography (OCT) and retinal photos for the diagnosis of cognitive alteration of neurodegenerative origin (all causes)	Up to 6 tot 12 weeks

Sponsor

Assistance Publique - Hôpitaux de Paris

Investigators

Principal Investigator: Emmanuel COGNAT, Dr. Cognitive Neurology Center, CMRR Paris Nord Ile-De France

General Publications

No publications available

Retina

Recruiting

United States

OCT Angiography and NRAI in Dementia

ClinicalTrials.gov ID NCT03761381

Sponsor Oregon Health and Science University
Information provided by David Huang, Oregon Health and Science University (Responsible Party)
Last Update Posted 2022-09-26

Brief Summary

The primary goals of this study are to use optical coherence tomography (OCT) angiography (blood vessel mapping) to:

1. Detect retinal blood vessels and blood flow changes in participants with dementia
2. Detect amyloid protein deposits in the retinas of participants with dementia

Official Title

Using Optical Coherence Tomography and Noninvasive Retinal Amyloid Imaging to Capture Retinal Changes Associated with Dementia

Conditions

Alzheimer Disease
Dementia
Mild Cognitive Impairment

Intervention/Treatment

- Device: Optical Coherence Tomography Angiography (OCTA) Imaging
- Device: Noninvasive Retinal Amyloid Imaging (NRAI)

Other Study ID Numbers

- IRB#00017045

Study Start (Actual)

2018-09-14

Primary Completion (Estimated)

2023-12

Study Completion (Estimated)

2024-12

Enrollment (Estimated)

20

Study Type

Observational

Study Contact

Name: Denzil Romfh, OD
Phone Number: 503-494-4351
Email: romfhd@ohsu.edu

Study Contact Backup

Name: Humberto Martinez, COT
Phone Number: 503-494-7712
Email: martinhu@ohsu.edu
United States
Oregon Locations

Portland, Oregon, United States, 97239
Recruiting
Oregon Health & Science University

Contact
Denzil Romfh, OD
503-494-4351 romfhd@ohsu.edu

Contact
Humberto Martinez, COT
503-494-7712 martinhu@ohsu.edu

Description
Inclusion Criteria for dementia subjects:

- Physician-confirmed diagnosis of probable Alzheimer's disease
- Mild dementia, as defined by a score of 20 or greater on the Mini-Mental State Exam, or a score of 15 or greater on the Montreal Cognitive Assessment, or a Clinical Dementia Rating Scale score of 1
- Age older than 55 years
- Able to comply with study procedures
- Corrected visual acuity at least 20/400 in either eye
- Has a legally authorized representative who can sign the study consent form and accompany the participant to the OCT study visit

Inclusion Criteria for dementia-free controls:

- Age older than 55 years
- Able to comply with study procedures
- Able to maintain stable fixation for OCT imaging
- Corrected visual acuity of at least 20/40 in either eye
- Dementia-free, as defined by a score of 24 or greater on the Mini-Mental Status Exam, or a score of 18 or greater on the Montreal Cognitive Assessment, or Clinical Dementia Rating of <1.0

Exclusion Criteria for both dementia and dementia-free subjects:

- Non-Alzheimer's disease related primary neurologic disease affecting the central nervous system (i.e., multiple sclerosis, Parkinson's disease)
- Evidence on ophthalmological exam within the last year of other ocular diseases or pathology that would confound the assessment of dementia (e.g., glaucoma, diabetic or hypertensive retinal disease, amblyopia, etc.)
- Media opacity such as cataract, corneal scar, or vitreous opacity that could interfere with retinal imaging
- Previous intraocular surgery except for uncomplicated cataract extraction with posterior chamber intraocular lens implantation
- Inability to maintain stable fixation for OCT imaging or provide informed consent
- Spherical equivalent refractive error greater than +3 or −7 diopters, or astigmatism magnitude of greater than 2 diopters.

- Diabetes for more than 10 years or hemoglobin A1C level of >10 within the 180 days prior to OCT scanning.
- Uncontrolled hypertension.: SBP >170 or DBP >100
- Arrhythmia: irregular pulse, or heart rate not between 50 and 110 beats per minute
- Pregnancy or breastfeeding.

Study Population

Dementia subjects will be recruited from the Layton Aging & Alzheimer's Disease Clinic at Oregon Health & Science University. Dementia-free subjects will be recruited from those currently being followed in the Layton Aging & Alzheimer's Disease Center Longitudinal Aging Study with MRI and amyloid PET imaging.

Ages Eligible for Study

55 Years and older (Adult, Older Adult)

Sexes Eligible for Study

All

Accepts Healthy Volunteers

Yes

Sampling Method

Probability Sample

Observational Model: Case–Control
Time Perspective: Prospective

Cohorts and interventions

Group/cohort	Intervention/treatment

Early dementia
This group will consist of adults with suspected dementia/ Alzheimer's disease. OCTA and NRAI data will be gathered in one study visit
	Device: optical coherence tomography angiography (OCTA) imaging
	  • Optical coherence tomography is a noninvasive imaging technology that provides cross-sectional images of tissues in micron-scale resolution. The angiography component of this device allows for the evaluation of blood vessels and blood flow changes in the eye. The Solix device with AngioVue software will be used to detect these blood vessels and flow changes as well as protein deposits in the retinal layers
	Device: noninvasive retinal amyloid imaging (NRAI)
	  • The spectralis will be used for NRAI. This system uses a special light source and optical filters to detect the fluorescence of amyloid proteins in the eye

Group/cohort	Intervention/treatment
Dementia-free controls This group will consist of adults without suspected dementia/ Alzheimer's disease. OCTA and NRAI data will be gathered in one study visit	Device: optical coherence tomography angiography (OCTA) Imaging • Optical coherence tomography is a noninvasive imaging technology that provides cross-sectional images of tissues in micron-scale resolution. The angiography component of this device allows for the evaluation of blood vessels and blood flow changes in the eye. The Solix device with AngioVue software will be used to detect these blood vessel and flow changes as well as protein deposits in the retinal layers Device: noninvasive retinal amyloid imaging (NRAI) • The spectralis will be used for NRAI. This system uses a special light source and optical filters to detect the fluorescence of amyloid proteins in the eye

Primary outcome measures

Outcome measure	Measure description	Time frame
Retinal amyloid protein detection	OCT and OCT angiography will be used to detect levels of amyloid protein deposits within the retina layers on the single enrollment visit only. An increase in protein detection is expected in the dementia group	1 day

Secondary outcome measures

Outcome measure	Measure description	Time frame
Decreased blood flow	OCT and OCT angiography will be used to detect blood flow in dementia vs. dementia-free controls. OCT and OCTA imaging will be taken on the single enrollment visit only. Decreased blood flow is expected in the dementia group	1 day
Decreased retinal perfusion	OCT and OCT angiography will be used to detect retinal perfusion deficits in dementia vs. dementia-free controls. OCT and OCTA imaging will be taken on a single enrollment visit only. Decreased retinal perfusion is expected in the dementia group	1 day

Sponsor

Oregon Health and Science University

Investigators

• Principal Investigator: David Huang, MD, PhD, Oregon Health and Science University

General Publications

No publications available

Retina

Recruiting

United States

Understanding Circadian Responses to Light in Persons with Mild Cognitive Impairment

ClinicalTrials.gov ID NCT05411822

Sponsor Icahn School of Medicine at Mount Sinai
Information provided by Mariana Figueiro, Icahn School of Medicine at Mount Sinai (Responsible Party)
Last Update Posted 2023-05-26

Brief Summary

The purpose of this research study is to investigate the relationship between light, the thickness of the pigment at the back of your eye, melatonin levels, and memory. The study will investigate whether changing light distribution pattern from "on-axis" (i.e., directed along the eye's visual axis to the fovea) to "off-axis" (i.e., directed on the periphery of the eye's visual axis) impact melatonin suppression in 24 mild cognitive impairment participants and 24 healthy, age-matched controls.

Detailed Description

Eligible enrolled subjects will be exposed to four different lighting conditions in addition to one dark control condition. There will be five study sessions and each one will last for 90 min and will be separated by 1 week. Subjects will collect three saliva samples, each one 30 min apart for melatonin levels during each study session.

Official Title

Understanding Circadian Responses to Light in Persons with Mild Cognitive Impairment and Alzheimer's Disease

Conditions

Mild Cognitive Impairment
Alzheimer Disease

Intervention/Treatment

- Device: Lighting Intervention Blue light
- Device: Lighting Intervention Green light

Other Study ID Numbers

- GCO 21-0400

Study Start (Actual)

2021-09-28

Primary Completion (Estimated)
2024-05-31

Study Completion (Estimated)
2024-05-31

Enrollment (Estimated)
48

Study Type
Interventional

Phase
Not Applicable

Study Contact
Name: Barbara Plitnick, BSN
Phone Number: 518366-9306
Email: barbara.plitnick@mountsinai.org
United States
New York Locations

Menands, New York, United States, 12204
Recruiting
Light and Health Research Center at Mount Sinai

Contact
Barbara Plitnick, BSN
518-366-9306 barbara.plitnick@mountsinai.org

Principal Investigator
Mariana Figueiro, PhD

Inclusion Criteria
- Mild cognitive impairment
- Age-matched healthy control
- Macular pigment density either <0.3 or >0.5

Exclusion Criteria
- Extensive brain vascular disease
- Parkinson's disease
- Bipolar disorder
- Seasonal depression
- Diabetes
- High blood pressure
- Obstructing cataracts
- Macular degeneration

- Diabetic retinopathy
- Use of melatonin supplements
- Use of beta blockers
- Use of sleep medications
- Use of antidepressant medication

Ages Eligible for Study
55 Years and older (Adult, Older Adult)

Sexes Eligible for Study
All

Accepts Healthy Volunteers
Yes

Primary Purpose: Treatment
Allocation: Randomized
Interventional Model: Crossover Assignment
Masking: Single (Participant)

Arms and interventions

Participant group/arm	Intervention/treatment
Experimental: lighting intervention blue Blue light (λ_{max} = 451 nm) on and off-axis	Device: lighting intervention blue light • Custom-made lighting fixture that will deliver the blue lighting intervention
Experimental: lighting intervention green Green light (λ_{max} = 522 nm) on and off axis	Device: lighting intervention green light • Custom-made lighting fixture that will deliver the green lighting intervention

Primary outcome measures

Outcome measure	Measure description	Time frame
Change in melatonin levels	Saliva samples will be collected for melatonin analysis	One sample will be collected every 30 min during each 90 min study session up to 5 weeks

Investigators
- Principal Investigator: Mariana Figueiro, PhD, Icahn School of Medicine

General Publications

No publications available

Retina

Enrolling by Invitation

United States

Can (Optical Coherence Tomography) Pictures of the Retina Detect Alzheimer's Disease at Its Earliest Stages?

ClinicalTrials.gov ID NCT06023446

Sponsor University of California, Davis
Information provided by University of California, Davis (Responsible Party)
Last Update Posted 2023-09-08

Brief Summary

Years before someone experiences the symptoms of Alzheimer's disease, a compound called amyloid beta (Aβ) builds up in the brain. Excess Aβ—directly or indirectly—causes many of the symptoms of Alzheimer's dementia. However, recent studies of the FDA-approved drugs lecanemab (Leqembi®) and aducanumab (Aduhelm®) indicate that removing Aβ from the brain does not stop Alzheimer's. Clearly, there are other problems that need to be fixed. The investigators are interested in the cause of Aβ buildup.

Non-neuronal support cells, called glia, keep neurons healthy by regulating water and nutrient levels for the neurons. They also help clear Aβ away from neurons. Maybe Aβ builds up when glia are unhealthy.

Glia are very hard to study in the brain. Luckily, the light-sensing part of the eye—the retina—is an extension of the brain. The investigators study glia in the retina to learn about glia in the brain.

To study retinal glia, the investigators take pictures of the retina with optical coherence tomography (OCT). OCT is safe, painless, and is used in many eye clinics to look at the structure of the retina. When the investigators take OCT pictures under a bright light, and compare those to OCT pictures collected in darkness, it gives the investigators information about glial function. In a study published in 2020 ("Optical coherence tomography reveals light-dependent retinal responses in Alzheimer's disease") the investigators showed that this functional OCT measurement was different in people with Alzheimer's dementia, compared to age-matched healthy adults.

The goal of this observational study is to compare people at a pre-dementia stage of Alzheimer's disease to people who do not have any signs at all of Alzheimer's disease. By "pre-dementia stage," the investigators mean people who are either cognitively normal, or have mild cognitive impairment, but have had a medical test that shows the chemical beginnings of Alzheimer's disease. Members of the comparison group will also be cognitively normal, or have mild cognitive impairment, but had a medical test that shows utterly no signs of Alzheimer's disease.

The main question this study, is whether functional OCT can tell these two groups apart. If so, that would:

- Help build the case for glial health being important in the earliest stages of Alzheimer's, which in turn could lead to new treatment strategies
- Suggest that functional OCT might be used as an early (pre-dementia) screening test for Alzheimer's disease

Participants will:

- Undergo a brief eye exam (the investigators will not dilate pupils for this study)
- Undergo a paper-and-pencil cognitive test (to help verify "normal" or "mild cognitive impairment" status)
- Take a brief one-page survey to collect demographic information (like age)
- Permit limited access to pre-existing medical or research records (to verify the presence/absence of the chemical beginnings of Alzheimer's disease)
- Take several OCT pictures of both eyes, in light and after 2 min of darkness (several rounds of images are taken)

The expectation is that all study procedures will fit within 2 h of 1 day.

Official Title
Illuminating Glial Dysfunction in Alzheimer's Disease With Optical Coherence
    Tomography

Conditions
Alzheimer Disease
Mild Cognitive Impairment

Intervention/Treatment
- Diagnostic Test: Optical Coherence Tomography

Other Study ID Numbers
- 1647468
- K08AG080178 (U.S. NIH Grant/Contract)

Study Start (Estimated)
2023-09-11

Primary Completion (Estimated)
2028-02-28

Study Completion (Estimated)
2028-02-28

Enrollment (Estimated)
100

Study Type
Observational

United States
California Locations

Sacramento, California, United States, 95816
University of California – Davis

Inclusion Criteria

- By clinician (or prior research) assessment, known to either be cognitively normal or have mild cognitive impairment
- Known Alzheimer's biomarker status. As of 2023-JUL, this must either be an amyloid PET scan or cerebrospinal fluid measurement of amyloid and tau levels
- NOTE: Although this is a study of the eyes, age-typical ocular/vision complaints are permissible, so long as the retina is thought to be healthy. This list of acceptable conditions includes most people who:

  - wear glasses
  - wear contacts
  - use over-the-counter eye drops
  - have mild cataracts (no surgery scheduled)
  - had cataracts removed
  - had eye muscle surgery (e.g., to correct eye misalignment)
  - had eyelid surgery (blepharoplasty)
  - are monitored by an ophthalmologist in case a problem with the retina develops (this is sometimes suggested for people with diabetes), but one or both retinas is/are thought to be completely healthy

Exclusion Criteria

- Pregnant women
- Prisoners
- Known *for both eyes* to have ocular health or vision abnormalities that are not age-typical. The list of unacceptable conditions includes most people who:

  - have a special corrective lens (glasses or contact lens) prescription with a sphere greater than 7
  - currently use prescription eye drops (e.g., for glaucoma)
  - have/had prior surgical treatment for a retinal problem (e.g., retinal detachment that required surgery)
  - have/had eye injections for age-related macular degeneration

Study Population

The investigators plan to recruit participants from:

- Participants (or prospective participants) in research on aging and cognition at the University of California—Davis.
- Patients (or prospective patients) of University of California—Davis neurologists.

Ages Eligible for Study

50 Years to 89 Years (Adult, Older Adult)

Sexes Eligible for Study

All

Accepts Healthy Volunteers
Yes

Sampling Method
Non-Probability Sample

Observational Model: Case–Control
Time Perspective: Cross-Sectional

Cohorts and interventions

Group/cohort	Intervention/treatment
Pre-dementia Alzheimer's By clinical assessment, these participants will either be cognitively normal or have mild cognitive impairment. They will enter the study having already completed some biomarker testing for Alzheimer's disease (e.g., amyloid PET, cerebrospinal fluid measurement amyloid, and tau). In this group, the biomarker testing is positive/abnormal, indicating a pre-dementia stage of Alzheimer's disease. In the language of the 2018 NIA-AA Research Framework, these participants have A+ in their AT(N) biomarker profile and are at clinical stages 1–3	Diagnostic test: optical coherence tomography • The retina is imaged using infrared light. Images collected in light are compared to those collected in darkness to extract information about function
No evidence of Alzheimer's By clinical assessment, these participants will either be cognitively normal or have mild cognitive impairment. They will enter the study having already completed some biomarker testing for Alzheimer's disease (e.g., amyloid PET, cerebrospinal fluid measurement amyloid, and tau). In this group, the biomarker testing is negative/normal. In the language of the 2018 NIA-AA Research Framework, these participants have A—in their AT(N) biomarker profile and are at clinical stages 1–3	Diagnostic test: optical coherence tomography • The retina is imaged using infrared light. Images collected in light are compared to those collected in darkness to extract information about the function

Primary outcome measures

Outcome measure	Measure description	Time frame
Light-dependent change in optical coherence tomography images	The investigators will obtain OCT B-scans of the span of the retina between the center of the optic disc and the fovea. Each B-scan will be spatially normalized and averaged to generate a profile of retinal reflectivity versus depth into the retina. Reflectivities in light will be compared to reflectivities in darkness. In both groups, the investigators expect that (1) over the photoreceptor inner and outer segments, the retina will be more reflective in light than in darkness, (2) in the more vitreal portions of the retina (the layers occupied by Müller glia), the retina will be slightly less reflective in light than in darkness The investigators expect group differences in that functional outcome. The largest group difference is expected near the exterior border of the Müller glia, where participants with a pre-dementia stage of Alzheimer's may have an exaggerated light-dependent change in reflectivity	Day 1 (less than 2 h)

Sponsor
University of California, Davis

Collaborators

- National Institute on Aging (NIA)

Investigators
No information provided

General Publications

- Bissig D, Zhou CG, Le V, Bernard JT. Optical coherence tomography reveals light-dependent retinal responses in Alzheimer's disease. Neuroimage. 2020 Oct 1;219:117022. https://doi.org/10.1016/j.neuroimage.2020.117022. Epub 2020 Jun 5.

Tears

Recruiting

Netherlands

The TearAD Study: Tear Biomarkers for Alzheimer's Disease (AD) Screening and Diagnosis (TearAD)

ClinicalTrials.gov ID NCT05655793

Sponsor Maastricht University Medical Center
Information provided by Maastricht University Medical Center (Responsible Party)
Last Update Posted 2022-12-19

Brief Summary
The goal of this observational longitudinal study is to investigate whether tear fluid is a noninvasive source of biomarkers for Alzheimer's disease. The main aim of the study is to evaluate diagnostic accuracy measures (sensitivity and specificity) of tear and retinal biomarkers to discriminate individuals with and without neurodegeneration.

Tear fluid from participants will be collected noninvasively with Schirmer's strips, which is a small paper strip placed in the lower eye lid for a maximum of 5 min. Additionally, standard, ultra-wide field and cross-sectional retinal images will be obtained.

Official Title
The TearAD Study: Tear Biomarkers for Alzheimer's Disease (AD) Screening and Diagnosis

Conditions

Alzheimer Disease

Intervention/Treatment
- Diagnostic Test: Tear Fluid collection (Schirmer's strip)
- Diagnostic Test: Retinal imaging

Other Study ID Numbers
- 20-033

Study Start (Actual)

2022-06-09

Primary Completion (Estimated)

2025-07-01

Study Completion (Estimated)

2025-07-01

Enrollment (Estimated)

200

Study Type

Observational [Patient Registry]

Study Contact

Name: Marlies Gijs, PhD
Phone Number: +31 (0)433872241
Email: marlies.gijs@mumc.nl

Study Contact Backup

Name: Nienke van de Sande, MSc
Phone Number: +31 (0)433875345
Email: nienke.van.de.sande@mumc.nl
Netherlands
Limburg Locations

Maastricht, Limburg, Netherlands, 6229 HX
Recruiting
Academic Hospital Maastricht

Contact

Marlies Gijs, PhD
marlies.gijs@mumc.nl

Noord-Holland Locations

Description

Inclusion Criteria (Healthy Controls)
- Available CSF, PET, CT, or MRI data to evaluate the presence/absence of neuro-degeneration (preferably within 1 year of inclusion in this study)
- Absence of cognitive complaints or treatment and did not seek help for cognitive complaints in the past
- MMSE score 26–30 at baseline
- Age >50 years
- Available for follow-up (up to 24 months)
- Written informed consent obtained and documented

Inclusion Criteria (Patients)
- Available CSF, PET, CT, or MRI data to evaluate the presence/absence of neuro-degeneration (preferably within 1 year of inclusion in this study)
- Available for follow-up (up to 24 months)
- Written informed consent obtained and documented
- Capable of giving informed consent themselves (MMSE score >17/30)

Exclusion Criteria (All Subjects)
- Ocular conditions that could influence tear biochemical parameters (including eye infection, eye inflammation, eye surgery within the last 28 days, or other acute eye conditions)
- Neurological or systemic chronic conditions known to interfere with retinal thickness (e.g., glaucoma, diabetes mellitus)
- Ocular conditions interfering with optical coherence tomography (OCT) quality/retinal thickness: e.g,. severe cataract, age-related macular degeneration, and glaucoma

Study Population
The patients will be selected from the population who visit the memory clinic and are willing to participate in scientific research.

Ages Eligible for Study
50 Years and older (Adult, Older Adult)

Sexes Eligible for Study
All

Accepts Healthy Volunteers
Yes

Sampling Method
Non-Probability Sample

Design Details
Observational Model: Cohort
Time Perspective: Prospective
Target Follow-up Duration: 2 Years
Biospecimen Retention: Samples with DNA
Biospecimen Description: The type of biospecimen that is retained is tear fluid collected with Schirmer's strips, CSF, and blood.

Cohorts and interventions

Group/cohort	Intervention/treatment
With neurodegeneration Includes patients with mild cognitive impairment and dementia	Diagnostic test: tear fluid collection (Schirmer's strip) • Tear fluid will be collected noninvasively from all participants with the use of Schirmer's strips, which are small paper strips placed in the lower eyelid for a maximum of 5 min Diagnostic test: retinal imaging • The retina from all participants will be visualized with the use of a standard (Clarus 700 Zeiss), ultra-wide field (Optos), and cross-sectional (Optical Coherence Tomography) retinal images
Without neurodegeneration Includes healthy controls and patients with subjective cognitive decline	Diagnostic test: tear fluid collection (Schirmer's strip) • Tear fluid will be collected noninvasively from all participants with the use of Schirmer's strips, which are small paper strips placed in the lower eyelid for a maximum of 5 min Diagnostic test: retinal imaging • The retina from all participants will be visualized with the use of a standard (Clarus 700 Zeiss), ultra-widefield (Optos), and cross-sectional (Optical Coherence Tomography) retinal images

Primary outcome measures

Outcome measure	Measure description	Time frame
Capability of tear biomarkers to discriminate individuals with neurodegeneration from those without neurodegeneration and assess the change in biomarker levels over time	Levels of tear biomarkers will be determined from the Schirmer's strips. The biomarker levels will be analyzed to see whether they can discriminate between people with and without neurodegeneration	Sampling done at $t = 0$, 1 and 2 years

Secondary outcome measures

Outcome measure	Measure description	Time frame
The difference in tear biomarker level between patients and controls, and between patient groups and how these differences change over time	Additional analysis to see whether tear biomarkers can also discriminate patients from controls and differences between patient groups	Sampling done at $t = 0$, 1 and 2 years
Correlation of biomarker levels in tears, blood, and cerebral spinal fluid (CSF)	This analysis will be done to determine the correlation between biomarkers of different body fluids	Baseline measurements ($t = 0$) will be used to determine correlation
Correlation between tear biomarkers and other ocular imaging biomarkers, as well as assessing the change of this correlation over time	The correlation between tear biomarkers and ocular imaging biomarkers (e.g., thickness of the retinal nerve fiber layer, retinal vasculature tortuosity) will be analyzed	Imaging done at $t = 0$, 1 and 2 years

Sponsor
Maastricht University Medical Center

Investigators
- Principal Investigator: Marlies Gijs, PhD, Maastricht University Medical Center

General Publications

No publications available

Telemedicine

Recruiting

New Jersey

Telerehabilitation Alzheimer's Disease Feasibility (TADF) (TADF)

ClinicalTrials.gov ID NCT04732182

Sponsor Bright Cloud International Corp
Information provided by Bright Cloud International Corp (Responsible Party)
Last Update Posted 2022-05-02

Brief Summary
This is a pilot RCT with equal arms: the experimental arm and (waitlist) control arm.

All participants will be in the early stages of Alzheimer's disease and on stable medication. They will all continue with this medication for their 6 months of participation.

The experimental group will add weekly training on the experimental device, 5 days a week for 8 weeks. Training will involve therapeutic games aimed primarily at the memory cognitive domain. All participants will receive weekly calls from a clinical coordinator and report on medication and overall health. Caregivers will also be enrolled so they support the trials.

Detailed Description
Participants will be randomized equally into an experimental group and a waitlist control group.

Experimental training will occur in the home and will last 8 weeks, each week having 5 sessions of therapeutic gameplay. Each session will start with vitals being measured and logged followed by motor and biosensor baselines. Subsequently, participants will play an increasing number of games, targeted at the major cognitive domains of memory (primarily), attention, and executive functions. Since sessions will increase in length, researchers expect that more than ten short games may eventually be played in each session.

This will be an ABAA protocol for the experimental group and a AABA protocol for the wait-list control group. Data will be sampled at baseline (A), during each rehabilitation session (B), mid-way through the study (at 2 months from baseline), and at the end of the study, at 4 months from baseline (A).

At the end of every 4 weeks of BrightGo training, the participant and caregiver will each fill out a custom subjective evaluation questionnaire.

Before crossover to the experimental protocol, participants in the waitlist group will continue with their daily routine and prescribed medication (which will be logged). After crossing over, they will add the BrightGo intervention to their daily routine.

Participants initially randomized to the experimental group will continue with daily routine and medication, and add the five sessions per week of experimental therapy. Once they cross over to the control arm after 8 weeks from the start, they will continue with their daily routine and prescribed medication (which will again be logged) for another 8 weeks.

All participants will receive a weekly call from the Clinical Coordinator to report on any health concerns, system issues, and medication use. Caregivers will also be enrolled so they support the trials.

Official Title

Telerehabilitation Combining Virtual Reality Adaptable Games and Drug Therapy for Early Alzheimer's Disease—Feasibility

Conditions

Alzheimer Disease
Healthy Aging

Intervention/Treatment

- Device: BrightGo cognitive training
- Drug: Standard of Care medication for early Alzheimer's Disease

Other Study ID Numbers

- Telerehab AD Feasibility
- R43AG065035 (U.S. NIH Grant/Contract)

Study Start (Actual)

2022-02-16

Primary Completion (Estimated)

2022-12-31

Study Completion (Estimated)

2023-02-28

Enrollment (Estimated)

14

Study Type

Interventional

Phase
Not Applicable

Study Contact
Name: Grigore C Burdea, PhD
Phone Number: 9084069334
Email: diplomatru@yahoo.com

Study Contact Backup
Name: Edward A Berde, MS
Phone Number: 7326400400
Email: ed@brightcloud.health
United States
New Jersey Locations

New Brunswick, New Jersey, United States, 08901-2066
Recruiting
Rutgers, The State University of New Jersey

Contact
Jasdeep S Hundal, PsyD
732-235-6332 jsh164@rwjms.rutgers.edu

Contact
Daniel Valdivia, B.S.
2013164424 djv85@gsbs.rutgers.edu

Principal Investigator
Jasdeep S Hundal, PsyD

North Brunswick, New Jersey, United States, 08902
Recruiting
Bright Cloud Int'l Corp

Contact
Grigore C Burdea, PhD
908-406-9334 diplomatru@yahoo.com

Contact
Edward A Berde, MS
732-640-0400 ed@brightcloud.health

Principal Invsestigator
Grigore C Burdea, PhD

Inclusion Criteria
- Age 65–85
- Diagnosis of early Alzheimer's (Montreal Cognitive Assessment [MoCA] score of 19–25)
- English speakers;

- Ability to actively move UE and to flex/extend fingers
- Stable on Aricept 10 mg daily intake or Exelon 9.5 mg patch medication
- Able to consent
- Living in the community in Central Jersey soas to facilitate researchers travel to home for system installation and/or repairs
- Living with a caregiver willing to support trials and be present during sessions
- Good upper extremity motor function, close to the full range of movement of arms and fingers

Exclusion Criteria
- Those younger than 65
- Participating in other research studies
- Severe visual impairments or legally blind
- Severe hearing loss or deafness
- Uncontrolled hypertension (>190/100 mmHg)
- Severe cognitive delay (MoCA <19)
- Non-English speakers
- Those unable to provide consent
- Unable to move arms and fingers, or with severe arthritis
- Severe propensity to simulation sickness
- Those who are not cooperative with the evaluations pre-study
- Those who cannot produce reliable scores on the neuropsychological pre-study assessment because they do not comprehend the test or have severe speech impairment
- Those not living with a caregiver willing to support trials, and a caregiver unwilling or unable to be present during sessions
- Those who are unwilling to allow home inspections to ascertain internet conditions in the home, to determine the best placement for the experimental system, to install and remove the system, and to provide repairs if needed

Ages Eligible for Study
65 Years to 85 Years (Older Adult)

Sexes Eligible for Study
All

Accepts Healthy Volunteers
Yes

Primary Purpose: Treatment
Allocation: Randomized
Interventional Model: Crossover Assignment
Interventional Model Description: Pilot RCT. Participants are randomized equally into the experimental group and a wait-list control group. Randomization will be based on a randomization table prepared by a contracted bio-statistician
Masking: Single (Outcomes Assessor)
Masking Description: Outcomes Assessor will not be told which group the participant is part of, so not be biased in evaluations

Arms and interventions

Participant group/arm	Intervention/treatment

Experimental: standard of care medication for early Alzheimer's disease and BrightGo device cognitive training
Participants randomized to the experimental group will have the standard of care and 8 weeks of experimental computer-based therapy on the device. Then they will cross over in the control arm. Total participation 4 months during which they will be on Aricept 10 mg daily or Exelon 9.5 mg patch
	Device: BrightGo cognitive training
	• Training on the BrightGo experimental device in the home
	• Other names:
	  – Gamification for cognitive therapy
	Drug: standard of care medication for early Alzheimer's disease
	• Participant takes 10 mg of Aricept daily or wears an Exelon 9.5 mg patch and is stable on one of these medications that were prescribed for diagnosis of early Alzheimer's disease
	• Other names:
	  – Aricept 10 mg daily or Exelon 9.5 mg patch

Other: standard of care medication for early Alzheimer's disease Waitlist controls will have standard of care only, before they cross over into the experimental group for BrightGo therapy. Total participation 4 months during which they will be on Aricept 10 mg daily or Exelon 9.5 mg patch	Drug: standard of care medication for early Alzheimer's disease • Participant takes 10 mg of Aricept daily or wears an Exelon 9.5 mg patch and is stable on one of these medications that were prescribed for diagnosis of early Alzheimer's disease • Other names: – Aricept 10 mg daily or Exelon 9.5 mg patch

Primary outcome measures

Outcome measure	Measure description	Time frame
Change in visual attention as measured by Neuropsychological Assessment Battery	Visual attention is measured with the dots test of the Neuropsychological Assessment Battery (NAB). This is a delayed recognition span paradigm, in which an array of dots is exposed for a brief period, followed by a blank interference page, followed by a new array with one additional dot. The subject needs to point to the "new" dot. The test was administered 3 times, minimum score 0 (none of the new dots found) to maximum 3 (all 3 new dots found)	At baseline, at 8 weeks from baseline (2 months), and at 16 weeks from baseline (4 months)
Controlled Oral Word Change in language and executive function as measured by the Association Test (CFL/PRW) of the Multilingual Aphasia Examination	Measure of language and executive function	At baseline, at 8 weeks from baseline (2 months), and at 16 weeks from baseline (4 months)

Outcome measure	Measure description	Time frame
Change in cognitive executive function assessment score	Trail Making Test B (TMT-B), NAB Executive Functioning Module. This is a timed test (seconds) with less time indicative of better executive function	At baseline, at 8 weeks from baseline (2 months), and at 16 weeks from baseline (4 months)
Change in verbal memory as measured by Hopkins Verbal Learning Test, Revised (HVLT-R)	Hopkins Verbal Learning Test, Revised (HVLT-R) is a measure of verbal memory. It provides a brief assessment of immediate recall, delayed recall, and delayed recognition. The subject is read a series of nouns in several categories, and they are asked to repeat these nouns by writing them on a piece of paper. The test is repeated three times, and each time the score is a count of how many nouns were remembered by the subject. The second phase of the test involves delayed recall, which is administered after about 20 min from the original test. Subject needs to write down all the nouns they remembered and these are counted. There is a maximum of 12 correct responses during delayed recall, so max score is 12	At baseline, at 8 weeks from baseline (2 months), and at 16 weeks from baseline (4 months)
Change in visuospatial memory as measured by Brief Visuospatial Memory Test, Revised (BVMT-R)	BVMT-R is a measure of visuospatial memory. In three Learning Trials, the subject views a stimulus page showing a geometric figure for 10 s, and there are 6 drawings presented. Then the subject is asked to draw as many of the figures as possible in their correct location on a page in the response booklet. A Delayed Recall Trial is administered after a 25-min delay. Last, a Recognition Trial, in which the respondent is asked to identify which of the 12 figures were included among the original geometric figures, is administered. Raw scores will be used, with higher numbers representing better outcomes	At baseline, at 8 weeks from baseline (2 months), and at 16 weeks from baseline (4 months)
Change in Beck Depression Inventory II (BDI II) score, a measure of depression severity	Participants' depression measures with higher scores indicating higher severity (worse mood). The score range is 0–63, with 0 indicating normal mood (no depression), 1–13 for minimal depression, 14–19 for mild depression, 20–28 for moderate, and 29–63 severe depression	At baseline, at 8 weeks from baseline (2 months), and at 16 weeks from baseline (4 months)

Secondary outcome measures

Outcome measure	Measure description	Time frame
Change in the participant's quality of life as measured by the Quality of Life in Alzheimer's Disease Patient Version (QoL-AD)	Questionnaire measures the quality of life for AD individuals (QoL-AD) The questionnaire has 13 items, each with 4 possible outcomes (poor 1 point to excellent 4 points). The score trance is 13 (worst) to 52 points representing the best outcome	At baseline, at 8 weeks from baseline (2 months), and at 16 weeks from baseline (4 months)
Functional Activities Questionnaire in Older Adults with Dementia	Questionnaire for AD patient independence in daily activities The questionnaire has 10 items, each with a 4 possible outcomes (normal 0 points to Dependent 3 points). The score trance is 0 (best outcome) to 30 points representing the worst outcome	At baseline, at 8 weeks from baseline (2 months), and at 16 weeks from baseline (4 months)
Test of Premorbid Functioning (TOPF)	The Advanced Clinical Solutions Test of Premorbid Functioning (TOPF) is a word reading test	At baseline, at 8 weeks from baseline (2 months), and at 16 weeks from baseline (4 months)
Controlled Oral Word Association Test (CFL/ PRW) of the Multilingual Aphasia Examination	Test measures language and executive function RANGE	At baseline, at 8 weeks from baseline (2 months), and at 16 weeks from baseline (4 months)
Categorical verbal fluency (Animal Naming)	Test measures language and executive function RANGE	At baseline, at 8 weeks from baseline (2 months), and at 16 weeks from baseline (4 months)
Quality of Life in Alzheimer's Disease (QoL-AD), Family Version	The Quality of Life in Alzheimer's Disease (QoL-AD) is comprised of 13 items (physical health, energy, mood, living situation, memory, family, marriage, friends, self as a whole, ability to do chores, ability to do things for fun, money, and life as a whole). Response options include 1 (poor), 2 (fair), 3 (good), and 4 (excellent) for a total score of 13–52, with higher scores indicating better QoL. Score range is 13 (worst outcome) to 52 (best outcome)	At baseline, at 8 weeks from baseline (2 months), and at 16 weeks from baseline (4 months)
Grasp strength (Jamar dynamometer)	Measure of sustained power grasping force. Three readings on a Jamar dynamometer are averaged. Higher values indicate more ability to grasp forcefully (a better outcome)	At baseline, at 8 weeks from baseline (2 months), and at 16 weeks from baseline (4 months)

Outcome measure	Measure description	Time frame
Pinch strength (Jamar pinch meter)	Measure of sustained pinch force. Three readings on a Jamar pinch meter are averaged. Higher values indicate more ability to pinch forcefully (a better outcome)	At baseline, at 8 weeks from baseline (2 months), and at 16 weeks from baseline (4 months)
Shoulder strength	Measure of deltoid muscle strength, measured using wrist weights. Higher values indicate more shoulder strength (a better outcome)	At baseline, at 8 weeks from baseline (2 months), and at 16 weeks from baseline (4 months)
Arm range of motion (goniometer)	Measure of upper extremity range of motion, measured using a mechanical goniometer. Higher values indicate more arm reach (a better outcome)	At baseline, at 8 weeks from baseline (2 months), and at 16 weeks from baseline (4 months)
Jebsen test of hand function	The timed battery of 7 simulated ADLs. Each task is timed with a stopwatch, with faster tack execution being a better outcome. The score range for each task is 1 s (best) to 180 s (worst—unable to execute a task).	At baseline, at 8 weeks from baseline (2 months), and at 16 weeks from baseline (4 months)
Cherokee test or independence in bimanual activities (CAHAI-9)	The test has nine simulated bimanual activities. Each task is scored in the amount of assistance needed to execute it, with a score range for each task of 1 (worst) to 7 (best). The total score range is 9 (worst) to 63 (best)	At baseline, at 8 weeks from baseline (2 months), and at 16 weeks from baseline (4 months)
University of Pennsylvania Smell Identification Test (UPSIT)	This test is a standardized measure of olfactory identification accuracy, done by scratching odor-generating special paper. The scents are released using a pencil. After each scent is released, the patient smells the level and detects the odor from the four choices. A higher score indicates better olfaction (better outcome). Minimum score is 0 and maximum score is 40	At baseline, at 8 weeks from baseline (2 months), and at 16 weeks from baseline (4 months)
Subjective evaluation of BrightGo system and therapy	Subjective evaluation on a 5-point Likert scale of the system and perceived benefits by the participant and by caregiver. The score range is 1 (worst outcome) to 5 (best outcome)	For experimental group test is at 4, and 8 weeks from baseline. For cross-over controlled test is at 12 and 16 weeks from baseline

Other outcome measures

Outcome measure	Measure description	Time frame
Cybersickness Susceptibility Questionnaire	Form used at screening post-consent to determine a participant's propensity for Determine propensity for simulation sickness. The questionnaire asks participants 13 general health and fitness questions (with yes/no answers) and to score 13 symptoms of cybersickness on a 5-point scale (0–4). The score range is 0 (best outcome—no likelihood of experiencing simulation sickness with the device) to 52 (worst outcome—certainty participant will experience severe simulation sickness)	At enrollment (20 min)
Montreal Cognitive Assessment (MoCA) to measure level of cognitive impairment	Used at screening post-consent to determine the level of cognitive impairment for participants. The form has a score range from 0 (worst) to 30 (best)—no cognitive impairments. The form will confirm a participant is in the score range of 19–25 range for early Alzheimer's disease	At enrollment (20 min)
Pulse	Hart rate measured with a medical meter	Before and after each of experimental session. For 3 months post-baseline for experimental group, or starting at 3 months from baseline for the control group. After cross over the control group will take pulse for 3 months
Blood pressure	Systolic and diastolic blood pressures, measured with a medical meter	Before and after each of experimental session. For 3 months post-baseline for the experimental group. For the control group it starts at 3 months from baseline for 3 more months
Game score	Scores obtained by participant for each game played on the BrightGo system are converted to percent, with 0% being the worst outcome and 100% being the best outcome	During each experimental session. For 2 months post-baseline for experimental group. For control group it starts at 3 months from baseline for 3 more months
Head movement	Obtained by participant Head Mounted Display during the BrightGo sessions	During each experimental session. For 2 months post-baseline for the experimental group. For the control group it starts at 3 months from baseline for 3 more months

Outcome measure	Measure description	Time frame
Biosensor measure (eyeblink)	Eye blink rates measured during game play	During each experimental session. For 2 months post-baseline for the experimental group. For the control group it starts at 3 months from baseline for 3 more months
Game difficulty	For each game played in an experimental session, the system stores its difficulty level. This has a range of 1 (lowest difficulty) to 16 (highest difficulty)	During each experimental session. For 2 months post-baseline for the experimental group. For the control group it starts at 3 months from baseline and for 3 more months
Biosensor measure (skin resistance)	During an experimental session, we store the skin resistance of the participant measured with a custom galvanic skin response system	During each experimental session. For 2 months post-baseline for the experimental group. For the control group it starts at 3 months from baseline and for 3 more months

Sponsor

Bright Cloud International Corp

Collaborators

- National Institute on Aging (NIA)
- Rutgers, The State University of New Jersey

Investigators

- Principal Investigator: Grigore C. Burdea, PhD, Bright Cloud International

General Publications

No publications available

Virtual Reality

Recruiting

Philippines

ImGTS for Patients with Behavioral and Psychological Symptoms of Dementia
(Phase 2)

ClinicalTrials.gov ID NCT06072014

Sponsor Augmented eXperience E-health Laboratory
Information   provided   by   Augmented   eXperience   E-health   Laboratory
    (Responsible Party)
Last Update Posted 2023-10-10

Brief Summary
The proposed research project aims to answer the question "Are immersive technology systems effective in the management and treatment of patients with BPSD?". This project is composed of three phases and the current study is the second phase. The phase 2 trial aims to create an immersive technology system for managing the behavioral and psychological symptoms of dementia and determine its clinical effectiveness, safety, usability, and acceptability among patients with mild to moderate Alzheimer's disease.

Official Title
Developing Immersive Gamification Technology Systems for the Management of
    Patients with Alzheimer's Disease with Behavioral and Psychological Symptoms
    of Dementia (Phase 2 Trial)

Conditions
Dementia Alzheimer's

Intervention/Treatment
- Other: Virtual reality

Other Study ID Numbers
- AXEL0003

Study Start (Actual)
2023-07-10

Primary Completion (Estimated)
2023-12

Study Completion (Estimated)
2023-12

Enrollment (Estimated)
30

Study Type
Interventional

Phase
Not Applicable

Study Contact
Name: Roland Dominic G. Jamora, MD, PhD
Phone Number: +639985438062
Email: rgjamora@up.edu.ph
Philippines
National Capital Region Locations

City Of Manila, National Capital Region, Philippines, 1000
Recruiting
University of the Philippines College of Allied Medical Professions Immersive
   Technology Laboratory

Contact
Maria Eliza R. Aguila, PhD
+639178212563 mraguila1@up.edu.ph

Inclusion Criteria
- Aged 60 years old or older
- Diagnosed with mild to moderate Alzheimer's dementia according to the National Institute of Neurological and Communicative Disorders and Stroke and the Alzheimer's Disease and Related Disorders Association (NINCDS-ADRDA) criteria
- Montreal Cognitive Assessment-Philippines (MOCA-P) score of 10–20 inclusive
- Neuropsychiatric Inventory (NPI-12) score 1–50 inclusive
- Reisberg Scale Stage 4–5 inclusive
- Stable dose of antidepressants for the past 6 weeks
- Stable dose of antipsychotics for the past 4 weeks
- Able to walk unassisted or with minimal assistance, with or without an assistive device
- No other explanation for the condition based on reasonable clinical diagnostics

Exclusion Criteria
- Have mild cognitive impairment (no dementia)
- Have MOCA-P score less than 10 or more than 20
- Other nonamnestic dementia syndromes
- Have receptive aphasia
- Have significant visual or hearing impairment
- Have an active psychiatric disorder prior to Alzheimer dementia diagnosis

- Had previous episodes of seizures, diagnosis of epilepsy, or intake of antiepileptic or seizure medications
- Have quadriplegia or paralysis of the dominant hand
- Have a history of motion sickness
- Experience claustrophobia
- Have a diagnosis of a terminal illness or a life expectancy of less than 1 year

Ages Eligible for Study
60 Years and older (Adult, Older Adult)

Sexes Eligible for Study
All

Accepts Healthy Volunteers
No

Primary Purpose: Supportive Care
Allocation: Randomized
Interventional Model: Parallel Assignment
Masking: Single (Outcomes Assessor)

Arms and interventions

Participant group/arm	Intervention/treatment
Experimental: head-mounted display (HMD) The HMD system uses a commercially available virtual headset, the Oculus/Meta Quest 2, which allows a user to view a virtual environment in 360° and to interact with the environment using hand-tracking technology (i.e., when a user's hand is projected into the virtual world to be used for interactions and gestures)	Other: virtual reality • A role-playing game with activities based on existing therapy activities (such as orientation therapy, reminiscence therapy, art therapy, and music therapy) that are used to manage behavioral and psychological symptoms of dementia
Experimental: semi-cave automatic virtual environment (semi-CAVE) The semi-CAVE system uses projectors and projector screens to provide a 270-degree view of the virtual environment. These projectors are connected to a powerful workstation (desktop computer), which uses HTC Vive trackers and base stations to track user movements and interactions	Other: virtual reality • A role-playing game with activities based on existing therapy activities (such as orientation therapy, reminiscence therapy, art therapy, and music therapy) that are used to manage behavioral and psychological symptoms of dementia

Primary outcome measures

Outcome measure	Measure description	Time frame
Incidence of behavioral and psychological symptoms of dementia will be assessed using the Neuropsychiatric Inventory-12	The NPI evaluates the degree and severity of BPSDs and the distress they cause the primary caregiver. Scores range from 0 to 120 where higher scores indicate greater psychiatric disturbance	Within 1 h after completion of the fourth session

Outcome measure	Measure description	Time frame
Incidence of virtual reality sickness symptoms will be assessed using the Virtual Reality Sickness Questionnaire	The VRSQ will measure a participant's experience with the following symptoms: general discomfort, fatigue, eye strain, difficulty focusing, headache, fullness of head, blurring of vision, dizziness (when eyes are closed), and vertigo. Symptoms will be rated on a 4-point scale: 0 or none, 1 or slight, 2 or moderate, and 3 or severe	Immediately after each intervention, within an hour of completion of the virtual reality game
Usability of the virtual reality intervention will be assessed using the System Usability Scale	The SUS is a 10-item questionnaire that is widely used in the evaluation of various kinds and aspects of technology. Each question has five response options ranging from "Strongly agree" to "Strongly disagree,", which has a corresponding number value. Each response is added and multiplied by 2.5 to obtain the final score that ranges from 0 to 100. A SUS score above 68 is considered above average	Immediately after each intervention, within an hour of completion of the virtual reality game

Secondary outcome measures

Outcome measure	Measure description	Time frame
Cognitive function will be assessed using MOCA-P	Montreal Cognitive Assessment-Philippines (MOCA-P) is a 30-item test that takes about 10–12 min to complete. The test measures different cognitive domains such as visuospatial/executive, naming, memory, attention, language, abstraction, and orientation	Within 1 h after completion of the fourth session
Cognitive function will be assessed using MMSE	The Mini-Mental State Exam (MMSE) is a 30-item test for cognitive function. It assesses attention, orientation, memory, registration, recall, calculation, language, and an individual's ability to draw a complex polygon	Within 1 h after completion of the fourth session
Cognitive function will be assessed using ADAS-Cog	The cognitive subscale of the Alzheimer's Disease Assessment Scale (ADAS-Cog) is an 11-item tool for the assessment of the following tasks: word recall, naming objects and fingers, commands, constructional praxis, ideational praxis, orientation, word recognition, and language	Within 1 h after completion of the fourth session
Activities of daily living will be assessed using ADCS-ADL	The Alzheimer's Disease Cooperative Study-Activities of Daily Living Inventory (ADCS-ADL) is a 24-item assessment of activities of daily living within the past 4 weeks	Within 1 h after completion of the fourth session
Health-related quality of life will be assessed using DEMQOL	The health-related quality of life for people with dementia (DEMQOL) is a 28-item self-report measure of quality of life specific for persons with mild-to-moderate dementia. It covers four dimensions of quality of life, namely, daily activities, memory, negative emotion, and positive emotion	Within 1 h after completion of the fourth session

Other outcome measures

Outcome measure	Measure description	Time frame
Acceptability	Acceptability will be measured among a small group of patients and their caregivers through an interview and a focus group discussion	Within 1 day of completing virtual reality experience

Sponsor

Augmented eXperience E-health Laboratory

Collaborators

No information provided

Investigators

- Principal Investigator: Veeda Michelle M. Anlacan, MD, University of the Philippines Manila

General Publications

- Anlacan, V.M.M. et al. (2023). Application Design for a Virtual Reality Therapy Game for Patients with Behavioral and Psychological Symptoms of Dementia. In: Krouska, A., Troussas, C., Caro, J. (eds) Novel & Intelligent Digital Systems: Proceedings of the 2nd International Conference (NiDS 2022). NiDS 2022. Lecture Notes in Networks and Systems, vol 556. Springer, Cham. https://doi.org/10.1007/978-3-031-17601-2_15.

Chapter 3
Treatment

Recruiting

United States

Understanding Circadian Responses to Light in Persons with Mild Cognitive Impairment

ClinicalTrials.gov ID NCT05411822

Sponsor Icahn School of Medicine at Mount Sinai
Information provided by Mariana Figueiro, Icahn School of Medicine at Mount Sinai (Responsible Party)
Last Update Posted 2023-05-26

Brief Summary
The purpose of this research study is to investigate the relationship between light, the thickness of the pigment at the back of your eye, melatonin levels, and memory. The study will investigate whether the changing light distribution pattern from "on-axis" (i.e., directed along the eye's visual axis to the fovea) to "off-axis" (i.e., directed on the periphery of the eye's visual axis) impacts melatonin suppression in 24 mild cognitive impairment participants and 24 healthy, age-matched controls.

Detailed Description
Eligible enrolled subjects will be exposed to four different lighting conditions in addition to one dark control condition. There will be five study sessions and each one will last for 90 min and will be separated by 1 week. Subjects will collect three saliva samples, each one 30 min apart for melatonin levels during each study session.

Official Title
Understanding Circadian Responses to Light in Persons With Mild Cognitive
Impairment and Alzheimer's Disease

Conditions
Mild cognitive impairment
Alzheimer's disease

Intervention/Treatment
- Device: Lighting intervention blue light
- Device: Lighting intervention green light

Other Study ID Numbers
- GCO 21-0400

Study Start (Actual)
2021-09-28

Primary Completion (Estimated)
2024-05-31

Study Completion (Estimated)
2024-05-31

Enrollment (Estimated)
48

Study Type
Interventional

Phase
Not applicable

Study Contact
Name: Barbara Plitnick, BSN
Phone Number: 518366-9306
Email: barbara.plitnick@mountsinai.org
United States
New York Locations

Menands, New York, United States, 12204
Recruiting
Light and Health Research Center at Mount Sinai

Contact
Barbara Plitnick, BSN
518-366-9306 barbara.plitnick@mountsinai.org

Principal Investigator
Mariana Figueiro, PhD

Eligibility Criteria
Description

Inclusion Criteria
- Mild-cognitive impairment
- Age-matched healthy control
- Macular pigment density either <0.3 or >0.5

Exclusion Criteria
- Extensive brain vascular disease
- Parkinson's disease
- Bipolar disorder
- Seasonal depression
- Diabetes
- High blood pressure
- Obstructing cataracts
- Macular degeneration
- Diabetic retinopathy
- Use of melatonin supplements
- Use of beta blockers
- Use of sleep medications
- Use of antidepressant medication

Ages Eligible for Study
55 Years and older (Adult, Older Adult)

Sexes Eligible for Study
All

Accepts Healthy Volunteers
Yes

Primary purpose: Treatment
Allocation: Randomized
Interventional Model: Crossover assignment
Masking: Single (participant)

Arms and interventions

Participant group/arm	Intervention/treatment
Experimental: lighting intervention blue Blue light (λ_{max} = 451 nm) on and off-axis	Device: lighting intervention blue light Custom-made lighting fixture that will deliver the blue lighting intervention
Experimental: lighting intervention green Green light (λ_{max} = 522 nm) on and off-axis	Device: lighting intervention green light Custom-made lighting fixture that will deliver the green lighting intervention

Primary outcome measures

Outcome measure	Measure description	Time frame
Change in melatonin levels	Saliva samples will be collected for melatonin analysis	One sample will be collected every 30 min during each 90 min study session up to 5 weeks

Sponsor
Icahn School of Medicine at Mount Sinai

Investigators
- Principal Investigator: Mariana Figueiro, PhD, Icahn School of Medicine

General Publications
No publications are available

Treatment

Recruiting

United States

Gamma Light and Sound Stimulation to Prevent Dementia in Cognitively Normal People at Risk for Alzheimer's Disease

ClinicalTrials.gov ID NCT05776641

Sponsor Massachusetts General Hospital
Information provided by Diane Chan, Massachusetts General Hospital (Responsible Party)
Last Update Posted 2023-09-13

Brief Summary
Alzheimer's disease (AD) is characterized by significant memory loss, toxic protein deposits (amyloid and tau) in the brain, and changes in the gamma frequency band on EEG. Gamma waves are important for memory, and in patients with AD, there are fewer gamma waves in the brain. The Tsai lab found that boosting gamma waves in AD mouse models using light and sound stimulation at 40 Hz not only reduced amyloid and tau in the brain but also improved memory. A light and sound device was developed for humans that stimulates the brain at 40 Hz and can be used safely at home. The goal of this study is to see if using this device can prevent dementia in people who are at risk for developing Alzheimer's disease.

Detailed Description
The investigators are recruiting participants aged 55+ with normal memory who have or had a close family member with Alzheimer's disease. Two hundred

participants will undergo a blood test and a subset will undergo an amyloid PET scan and only 50 participants who have cerebral amyloid deposits will continue in the study. Neither the participant nor the investigators will know whether the participant is receiving sham or active stimulation. Participants will use the device for 12 months at home, for 60 min each day when they are awake. Participants will come to the Massachusetts General Hospital in Boston for 4–6 visits: before starting the stimulation, at 6 months, and after 12 months of usage. The participants will undergo PET scans, MRI, EEG, blood tests, memory tests, and questionnaires at each visit to monitor progress. In addition, people may elect to allow us to study their cerebral spinal fluid. Participants will also wear a "fitbit" like watch to monitor sleep and activity throughout the study. The goal of this study is to evaluate whether stimulation with our device at 40 Hz will reduce AD pathology in the brain.

Official Title
Prevention of Alzheimer's disease Using Gamma Entrainment

Conditions
Alzheimer disease
Family members

Intervention/Treatment
- Device: GENUS

Other Study ID Numbers
- 2021P002885

Study Start (Estimated)
2023-10-01

Primary Completion (Estimated)
2025-05

Study Completion (Estimated)
2026-05

Enrollment (Estimated)
200

Study Type
Interventional

Phase
Not applicable

Study Contact
Name: Kenji Aoki, BA
Phone number: 617-258-7723
Email: kenji292@mit.edu

Study Contact Backup
Name: Gabrielle de Weck, BS
Phone number: 617-258-7723
Email: gdeweck@mit.edu
United States
Massachusetts Locations

Boston, Massachusetts, United States, 02114
Recruiting
Massachusetts General Hospital

Contact
Kenji Aoki, BA
617-258-7723 kenji292@mit.edu

Contact
Gabrielle de Weck, BS
617-258-7723 gdeweck@mit.edu

Principal Investigator
Diane Chan, MD PhD

Eligibility Criteria
Description

Inclusion Criteria
- Between 55 and 90 years of age, inclusive
- Immediate family history of Alzheimer's disease
- Mini-Mental State Exam (MMSE) score of 27 or greater at baseline or expected score range for cognitively normal adjusted for the education level
- Clinical Dementia Rating Global Score of 0 at baseline
- Delayed Recall score on the Logical Memory IIa subtest of 8–15 at baseline or expected score range for cognitively normal adjusted for education level
- Low serum amyloid levels at baseline
- Elevated fibrillar amyloid using 11C PiB PET at baseline between 20 and 70 CL
- Willing and able to undergo MRI brain and PET brain scans
- Adequate visual and auditory acuity to allow for neuropsychological testing
- Able to comply with neuropsychological testing and other study procedures in the opinion of site PI
- Willing and able to complete baseline assessments, and willing to participate in 13-month study protocol
- Willing to provide blood samples at specified time points. Willing to consider contributing CSF samples at specified timepoints, if asked

Exclusion Criteria

- MRI contraindications, such as the presence of pacemakers, aneurysm clips, artificial heart valves, ear implants, metal fragments, or foreign objects in the eyes, skin, or body
- High myopia <-7 diopters, or untreated cataracts that affect vision
- Any significant systemic illness or unstable medical condition that could lead to difficulty complying with the study protocol
- For subjects agreeing to undergo lumbar punctures, a history of bleeding disorders or laboratory results indicating low platelet levels are exclusionary for the procedure
- Concomitant medications:

  - Treatment with NMDA antagonists
  - For subjects undergoing lumbar puncture, current use of warfarin or similar anti-coagulants is exclusionary for the procedure

- Clinical conditions:

  - History of seizure or medical diagnosis of epilepsy
  - Female subjects who are pregnant or currently breastfeeding
  - History of severe allergic or anaphylactic reactions
  - Longstanding premorbid history (i.e., longer than 10 years) of alcohol or substance abuse with continuous abuse up to and including the time that the symptoms leading to clinical presentation developed
  - Neurodegenerative disorder associated with cognitive impairment
  - Renal disease

- MR imaging findings such as stroke, tumor, and leukoencephalopathy that could preclude meaningful analyses of clinical and imaging data in the opinion of the site PI, such as:

  - Severe leukoencephalopathy seen on MRI
  - Relevant structural abnormality (i.e., normal pressure or obstructive hydrocephalus, hypoxic ischemic lesions, hemorrhages, tumors, and malformations)
  - Cerebral amyloid angiopathy, evidenced by $T2^*$ or other susceptibility weighted-MRI

- Laboratory findings, if known (study does not perform testing) suggestive of systemic illness such as renal disease
- Site investigator's discretion, if s/he feels the subject cannot complete sufficient key study procedures. Exceptions to these guidelines may be considered on a case-by-case basis at the discretion of the Project Director

Ages Eligible for Study
55 Years to 90 Years (adult, older adult)

Sexes Eligible for Study
All

Accepts Healthy Volunteers
Yes

Primary purpose: Prevention
Allocation: Randomized
Interventional model: Parallel assignment
Masking: Quadruple (participant care provider investigator outcomes assessor)

Arms and interventions

Participant group/arm	Intervention/treatment
Active comparator: active GENUS light and sound The device is a light and sound device that delivers light stimulation using light-emitting diodes (LED) and sound stimulation through a speaker, with a centrally mounted tablet that plays videos for entertainment. The device will be positioned on an easel such that the tablet is at the eye level with the participant while they are sitting 5 ft away. The active device delivers light and sound at a 40 Hz rate	Device: GENUS • Participants will use the GENUS light and sound device at home for 60 min daily for 12 months
Sham comparator: sham GENUS light and sound The device is the same as the active device but it delivers light and sound at different frequencies	Device: GENUS • Participants will use the GENUS light and sound device at home for 60 min daily for 12 months

Primary outcome measures

Outcome measure	Measure description	Time frame
Changes in brain amyloid deposition over the study period, as measured by PiB PET	The investigators will evaluate changes from baseline in amyloid deposition by using Pittsburgh compound B (PiB) PET, which is a standard for AD trial biomarkers, to assess progression towards AD with active or sham treatment	Baseline of 12 months

Secondary outcome measures

Outcome measure	Measure description	Time frame
Changes in brain tau deposition	The investigators will evaluate changes from baseline in tau deposition by using MK-6240 PET	Baseline to 12 months
Changes in brain structure using structural MRI	The investigators will evaluate changes in brain structure using structural MRI. Preliminary data show prevention of brain atrophy after 3 months of GENUS as measured by ventricular dilation and hippocampal volume. Using structural MRI, the investigators will evaluate brain volume, cortical thickness, and ventricular volume	Baseline to 12 months
Changes in brain electrical activity	The investigators will evaluate brain electrical activity using longitudinal EEG (i.e., gamma band power)	Baseline to 12 months
Changes in brain connectivity by functional MRI	The investigators will evaluate connectivity using resting-state functional MRI to assess changes in brain networks (i.e., default mode network)	Baseline to 12 months
Changes to rest-activity parameters using actigraphy	Actigraphy will be used to evaluate rest-activity parameters (i.e., interdaily stability)	Baseline to 12 months

Outcome measure	Measure description	Time frame
Changes in blood biomarkers of AD	Changes in Alzheimer's blood-based biomarkers (e.g., plasma Aβ42/Aβ40 ratio, Aβ42, Aβ40, p-tau, and neurofilament light) assessed by longitudinal blood sample collection	Baseline to 12 months
Compliance of usage as measured by timestamp tracking and eye-tracking technology	The device contains both a time counter to track 'on time' and a camera that records images for eye-tracking, to quantitatively determine compliance with looking directly at the device. This method also quantifies whether the subjects are awake for the duration of treatment. Previous work with healthy older adults and a small cohort of mild AD patients has had 90% compliance	Baseline to 12 months
Change from baseline in CSF levels of amyloid and tau	Lumbar puncture and CSF collection will be optional for participants but will be informative as to the investigator's hypothesized mechanisms of clearance	Baseline to 12 months

Other outcome measures

Outcome measure	Measure description	Time frame
Changes in CSF flow, as measured by BOLD fMRI	The investigators will evaluate changes from baseline in CSF flow by using BOLD fMRI. CSF flow has been linked to amyloid clearance from the brain, and brain waste clearance mechanisms such as blood vessel dilation and increased glymphatic drainage are activated after 40-Hz light and sound stimulation in our preliminary mouse studies	Baseline to 12 months
Change from baseline in the integrity of white matter tracks and myelination as measured by diffusion MR imaging	It is hypothesized that neuromodulation causes changes in synaptic plasticity. The investigators will evaluate plasticity and structural measures of connectivity using diffusion imaging techniques	Baseline to 12 months
Changes in performance on memory tasks, particularly those that are reliant on visual or auditory pathways, using a neuropsychological test battery	The investigators will evaluate changes from baseline in performance on memory tasks using a comprehensive neuropsychological battery designed to evaluate pre-clinical AD populations. Preliminary data showed that 3 months of treatment in mild AD patients led to improved performance on an associative memory task	Baseline to 12 months
Change from baseline in gamma oscillations as measured by EEG	Magnetoencephalogram studies done in AD patients show decreases in endogenous gamma synchronization. We will measure induced gamma entrainment using the GENUS device with EEG	Baseline to 12 months
Change from baseline in sleep	The investigators will evaluate sleep quality using the Pittsburgh Sleep Quality Index	Baseline to 12 months
Change from baseline in activity levels	The investigators will evaluate activity levels using actigraphy	Baseline to 12 months
Incidence of adverse events	Adverse events as a result of GENUS stimulation will be reported	Baseline to 12 months

Sponsor
* Massachusetts General Hospital

Collaborators
* Massachusetts Institute of Technology

Investigators
* Principal Investigator: Diane Chan, MD PhD, Massachusetts General Hospital

General Publications
No publications available

Treatment

Recruiting

United States

Chronic Treatment of Alzheimer's Disease by Gamma Light
and Sound Therapy

ClinicalTrials.gov ID NCT05655195

Sponsor Massachusetts Institute of Technology
Information provided by Massachusetts Institute of Technology (Responsible Party)
Last Update Posted 2023-09-28

Brief Summary
Alzheimer's disease (AD) is characterized by significant memory loss, toxic protein
deposits (amyloid and tau) in the brain, and changes in the gamma frequency band
on EEG. The investigator's lab found that boosting gamma waves in AD mouse
models using light and sound stimulation at 40 Hz not only reduced amyloid and tau
in the brain but also improved memory. The investigators developed a light and
sound device for humans that stimulates the brain at 40 Hz that can be used safely
at home. For the present study, 50 participants with mild Alzheimer's disease will
be enrolled and will use this light and sound device at home daily for 6 months.
Investigators will measure changes in brain waves with EEG, blood biomarkers,the
microbiome via fecal samples, functional and structural MRI scans, memory and
cognitive testing, and questionnaires at three in-person visits throughout the study.
After the 6-month time point, participants will have the option of continuing in the
study for 1 additional year and completing an 18-month study visit. This study will
provide critical insight into extended therapy involving noninvasive 40 Hz sensory
stimulation as a possible therapeutic strategy for mild to moderate Alzheimer's
disease.

Detailed Description

Alzheimer's disease (AD) is characterized by significant memory loss, toxic protein deposits (amyloid and tau) in the brain, and changes in the gamma frequency band on EEG. Gamma waves are important for memory, and in patients with AD, there are fewer gamma waves in the brain. The investigator's lab found that boosting gamma waves in AD mouse models using light and sound stimulation at 40 Hz not only reduced amyloid and tau in the brain but also improved memory. The investigators developed a light and sound device for humans that stimulates the brain at 40 Hz that can be used safely at home. The investigators also developed a vibrating device for humans that stimulates the brain at 40 Hz via tactile stimulation. The investigators want to see if using these devices can prevent dementia in people who are at risk for developing Alzheimer's disease.

The investigators are recruiting 50 participants who have been diagnosed with Alzheimer's disease to participate in this study. There will be a small cohort of 4 early-onset AD participants aged 50–65, and the rest will be diagnosed with typical AD and aged 65+. It will take place at the Massachusetts Institute of Technology in Cambridge, MA, and will last 6 months with 3 required visits to the institution: the first at baseline, the second at 3 months, and the last after 6 months. Visits will include blood tests, fecal samples, EEG (using light, sound, and tactile stimulation), MRI, memory and cognitive tests, and questionnaires to monitor progress. Participants will take home a gamma light and sound device to use daily as well as a "Fitbit" type of watch to wear to track sleep patterns. Half of the participants will receive sham treatment, meaning they will use the investigators' device but the light and sound will not be set at 40 Hz. The other half will receive the same device but it will be set to stimulate the brain with 40 Hz light and sound. Neither the participant nor the investigators will know whether the participant is receiving sham or active stimulation. Participants will use the device for 6 months at home, for 60 min each day when they are awake. After 6 months, participants will have the option of continuing in the study for 1 additional year, during which time they will be guaranteed the 40 Hz active treatment, regardless of their original group assignment. For this additional year, participants will continue to use the device for 60 min every day, and they will come in for a final visit to MIT at the 18-month time point.

The purpose of this study is to determine whether gamma entrainment through noninvasive 40 Hz sensory stimulation is possible in those with AD, and whether functional connectivity in their brain and molecular biomarkers of AD will change after 6 months of daily treatment with the investigators' light and sound device. The treatment's impact on the microbiome, cognition, and daily sleep and activity will also be measured. This study will provide critical insight into extended therapy involving noninvasive 40 Hz sensory stimulation as a possible therapeutic strategy for mild to moderate Alzheimer's disease.

Official Title

Chronic Treatment of Alzheimer's Disease With Gamma Frequency Stimulation

Conditions
Alzheimer's disease
Alzheimer's disease, Early Onset
Alzheimer's disease, Late Onset
Alzheimer's disease (Incl Subtypes)
Alzheimer's
Alzheimer's disease

Intervention/Treatment
- Device: GENUS device (Active Settings)
- Device: GENUS device (sham settings)

Other Study ID Numbers
- 2206000685

Study Start (Actual)
2022-12-14

Primary Completion (Estimated)
2024-09-01

Study Completion (Estimated)
2024-09-01

Enrollment (Estimated)
50

Study Type
Interventional

Phase
Not Applicable

Study Contact
Name: Gabrielle De Weck, BS
Phone Number: 617-258-7723
Email: gdeweck@mit.edu

Study Contact Backup
Name: Megan Colburn, MS
Phone Number: 617-258-7723
Email: mcolburn@mit.edu
United States
Massachusetts Locations

Cambridge, Massachusetts, United States, 02142
Recruiting
Massachusetts Institute of Technology

Contact
Gabrielle De Weck, BS
617-258-7723 gdeweck@mit.edu

Contact

Megan Colburn, MS

617-258-7723 mcolburn@mit.edu

Description

Inclusion Criteria

Subjects may be enrolled in the study if they meet all of the following criteria:

- Subject is between the age of 50 and 100
- Subject must have mild Alzheimer's disease with a Mini Mental State Exam (MMSE) score of 19–26
- Subject is willing to sign an informed consent document
- If subject is deemed to not have capacity to sign the informed consent, then he/she will need a legally authorized representative to provide surrogate consent
- Able to complete the first month of at home stimulation at their primary residence. If subjects plan to spend more than 1 week away from their primary residence during the trial, then their inclusion must be assessed by the research team

Exclusion Criteria

Subjects who meet any of the following conditions will not be enrolled in the study:

- Subjects who do not have healthcare
- Subjects who are currently taking amyloid-reducing therapy
- Subjects who have >3 microbleeds/microhemmorhages in their brain
- Active treatment on a dosage of one or more psychiatric agents (e.g., antidepressants, antipsychotics, etc.) for LESS THAN 3 months (a stable dose for greater than or equal to 3 months is ok)
- Subjects who are being treated with N-methyl-D-aspartate (NMDA) receptor antagonists (e.g., Memantine)
- Subjects on medications that lower seizure threshold such as ellbutrin, ciprofloxacin, and levofloxacin.
- Subjects with a history of seizure or epilepsy within the past 24 months
- Subjects with clinically significant suicide risk and/or suicide attempt in the past 1 year
- Subjects with behavioral problems such as aggression/agitation/impulsivity that might interfere with their ability to comply with protocol
- Active treatment with one or more anti-epileptic agents
- Subjects who have had a stroke within the past 24 months
- Subjects who have had eye surgery in the last 3 months or are scheduled to have eye surgery in the next 6 months (during the study)
- Subjects diagnosed with migraine headache
- Subjects who have an active implantable medical device including but not limited to implantable cardioverter defibrillator (ICD), deep brain stimulator (DBS), cardiac pacemaker, and/or sacral nerve stimulator
- Subjects who have profound hearing or visual impairment
- Subjects who have a life expectancy of less than 2 years

- Subjects who are pregnant
- Current or past history of any neurological disorder other than dementia, such as epilepsy, stroke, progressive neurologic disease (e.g., multiple sclerosis) or intracranial brain lesions; and history of previous neurosurgery or head trauma that resulted in residual neurologic impairment

Ages Eligible for Study
50 Years to 100 Years (Adult, Older Adult)

Sexes Eligible for Study
All

Accepts Healthy Volunteers
Yes

Primary Purpose: Treatment
Allocation: Randomized
Interventional Model: Parallel Assignment
Masking: Double (Participant Investigator)

Arms and interventions

Participant group/arm	Intervention/treatment

Active comparator: Alzheimer's active arm
Exposure to active sensory stimulation (40 Hz) for 60 min daily for the length of the trial (6 months)
	Device: GENUS device (active settings)
	• Participants in the active, experimental group will use the GENUS devices configured to active (40 Hz) setting for 60 min daily for 6 months
	• Other Names:
	  – Gamma Frequency Stimulation
	  – Light and Sound Stimulation

Sham comparator: Alzheimer's control arm
Exposure to control stimulation (sham) for 60 min daily for the length of the trial (6 months)
	Device: GENUS device (sham settings)
	• Participants in the control group will use the GENUS devices configured to the sham settings for 60 min daily for 6 months
	• Other Names:
	  – Gamma frequency stimulation
	  – Light and sound stimulation

Primary outcome measures

Outcome measure	Measure description	Time frame
Feasibility of gamma frequency stimulation as assessed by a change of the gamma frequency waves during EEG	Feasibility of gamma frequency stimulation in subjects with AD will be assessed by analyzing the EEG data from each subject as they undergo gamma light, sound, and tactile stimulation. Investigators will look for a sign of change in gamma frequency waves and determine the percent of subjects who show this change. This change will be assessed through FFT analyses on the EEG data in MATLAB, which looks at the different frequencies that were present during the EEG session	Immediately after completing the stimulation at baseline, month 3, and month 6 visits

Outcome measure	Measure description	Time frame
Baseline incidence of stimulation-related adverse symptoms and side effects as assessed by post-stimulation questionnaires	Tolerability and safety of the gamma frequency stimulation will be assessed by using a questionnaire asking for the subjects' overall experience with the stimulation and denoting any adverse effects. Subjects will be asked specifically about headaches, light headedness, nausea, dizziness, dry eye, eye strain, light sensitivity, ringing in ears, and any other symptoms they are experiencing	Immediately after the completion of the stimulation at baseline
Mid-point incidence of stimulation-related adverse symptoms and side effects as assessed by post-stimulation questionnaires	Tolerability and safety of gamma frequency stimulation will be assessed by using a questionnaire asking for the subjects' overall experience with the stimulation and denoting any adverse effects. Subjects will be asked specifically about headaches, light headedness, nausea, dizziness, dry eye, eye strain, light sensitivity, ringing in ears, and any other symptoms they are experiencing	Immediately after the completion of the stimulation at month 3
Endpoint incidence of stimulation-related adverse symptoms and side effects as assessed by post-stimulation questionnaires	Tolerability and safety of gamma frequency stimulation will be assessed by using a questionnaire asking for the subjects' overall experience with the stimulation and denoting any adverse effects. Subjects will be asked specifically about headaches, light headedness, nausea, dizziness, dry eye, eye strain, light sensitivity, ringing in ears, and any other symptoms they are experiencing	Immediately after the completion of the stimulation at the end of the trial—month 6 timepoints
Change in stimulation-related adverse symptoms and side effects as assessed by post-stimulation questionnaires	Tolerability and safety of gamma frequency stimulation will be assessed by using a questionnaire asking for the subjects' overall experience with the stimulation and denoting any adverse effects. Subjects will be asked specifically about headaches, light headedness, nausea, dizziness, dry eye, eye strain, light sensitivity, ringing in ears, and any other symptoms they are experiencing	During weekly phone calls throughout the 6-month trial period
Changes in functional brain connectivity as measured by changes in brain white matter on functional MRI scans	Exploratory measure to check if there are changes in functional brain connectivity after 6 months of daily treatment with the light and sound device. Diffusion tensor imaging (DTI) will be used to test the connectivity and blood flow of the brain by identifying major white matter tracts. These data will be collected at baseline, month 3, and month 6 for each subject, and change will be determined by comparing these time points	At baseline, month 3, and month 6 visits during MRI sessions
Changes in functional brain connectivity as measured by changes in blood-oxygen-level-dependent (BOLD) signals on functional MRI scans	Exploratory measure to check if there are changes in functional brain connectivity after 6 months of daily treatment with the light and sound device. BOLD (blood-oxygen-level-dependent) imaging will be used to determine how regions are communicating and activating together via blood flow. These data will be collected at baseline, month 3, and month 6 for each subject, and change will be determined by comparing these time points	At baseline, month 3, and month 6 visits during MRI sessions

Outcome measure	Measure description	Time frame
Changes in gamma entrainment, as measured by the change in response to 40 Hz frequency during EEG sessions	Exploratory measure to check if there are changes in gamma entrainment after months of daily treatment with the light and sound device. Gamma entrainment during light and sound stimulation will also be assessed using EEG and FFT analyses in MATLAB to determine the degree to which the brain is responding to the 40 Hz frequency. These data will be collected at baseline, month 3, and month 6 for each subject, and change will be determined by comparing these time points	At baseline, month 3, and month 6 visits during EEG sessions
Changes in molecular biomarkers in AD as measured by RNA sequencing data, particularly those related to inflammation and amyloid levels	Exploratory measure to check if there are changes in molecular biomarkers of AD (based on RNA sequencing data) as a result of 6 months of daily treatment with the light and sound device. RNA information will be extracted from the subjects' blood samples at the baseline and month 6 visits. RNA sequencing of this blood is included based on previous transcriptomic analysis of peripheral leukocytes that showed that inflammation-related genes are related to neurodegenerative diseases such as AD. Change will be determined by comparing RNA-sequencing data between baseline and month 6 (the beginning and end of the trial)	Immediately after the blood draw at baseline and month 6 visits

Secondary outcome measures

Outcome measure	Measure description	Time frame
Changes in the microbiome as measured by fecal samples	At baseline and month 6, subjects will produce a fecal sample and hand it off to study staff for storage and sample processing using the QIAamp PowerFecal Pro DNA Kit (Qiagen). Data will then be analyzed using the Divisive Amplicon Denoising Algorithm 2 (DADA2) pipeline, which will provide gut microbial composition in the different experimental groups. Pipeline outputs involve principal component analyses, and a custom in-house script will be used to make statistical comparisons. Change will be assessed by comparing the fecal sample analyses between baseline and month 6	Immediately after fecal sample collection at baseline and month 6
Changes in cognitive performance as assessed by scores on an Alzheimer's cognitive testing battery	Exploratory measure to check if there is any change in cognitive performance as a result of 6 months of daily sessions with the light and sound device. Alzheimer's testing battery will be administered at baseline, month 3, and month 6 visits, and change will be determined by comparing cognitive performance (via standardized scores) at these three time points. These tests measure a variety of cognitive abilities, including attention, different types of memory, processing speed, visual acuity, and more	Immediately after completion of cognitive batteries at baseline, month 3, and month 6 visits

Outcome measure	Measure description	Time frame
Changes in sleep/wake patterns, as measured by actigraph watch analyses	Subjects will be expected to wear a GTX9 actigraph watch daily to record activity and sleep/wake patterns throughout the 6 months of the trial. This watch is like a regular wristwatch, but it records daily activity and patterns through light and movement. The subject will be given their watch ~2 weeks before the trial start date, and they will bring it in with them at baseline, month 3, and month 6 visits so researchers can download their data to analyze their length and quality of sleep, as well as their other circadian rhythms and patterns throughout each day. Change will be assessed by comparing actigraph data between baseline, month 3, and month 6, as the subject progress throughout the trial	Immediately after actigraph data download at baseline, month 3, and month 6

Sponsor

Massachusetts Institute of Technology

Investigators

- Principal Investigator: Li Huei Tsai, PhD, Massachusetts Institute of Technology

General Publications

No publications available

Treatment

Recruiting

United States

Vestibular Therapy in Alzheimer's Disease

ClinicalTrials.gov ID NCT03799991

Sponsor: Johns Hopkins University
Information provided by Johns Hopkins University (Responsible Party)
Last Update Posted 2022-12-14

Brief Summary

Nearly two out of three patients with Alzheimer's disease (AD) experience problems with balance and mobility, which places such patients at increased risk of falling. The vestibular (inner ear balance) system plays an important role in balance stability, and vestibular therapy (VT) is well known to improve balance function in healthy older adults. In this study, the investigators will conduct a first-in-kind randomized clinical trial to evaluate whether vestibular therapy improves reduces falls in patients with AD, in whom this treatment has never been studied.

Official Title
Vestibular therapy in Alzheimer's Disease

Vestibular diseases
Vestibular Alzheimer's disease

Intervention/Treatment
- Behavioral: Vestibular physical therapy
- Behavioral: Active control

Other Study ID Numbers
- IRB00273752

Study Start (Actual)
2021-03-01

Primary Completion (Estimated)
2024-06-30

Study Completion (Estimated)
2024-06-30

Enrollment (Estimated)
100

Study Type
Interventional

Phase
Not Applicable

Study Contact
Name: Yuri Agrawal, MD
Phone Number: 4105023107
Email: yagrawa1@jhmi.edu
United States
Maryland Locations

Baltimore, Maryland, United States, 21287
Recruiting
Johns Hopkins University School of Medicine

Contact
Yuri Agrawal

Principal Investigator
John Carey, MD

Inclusion Criteria
- Diagnosis of AD based on the National Institute on Aging-Alzheimer Association 2011 criteria that is mild-moderate (CDR = 0.5–2)
- Age ≥60 years
- Vestibular loss is defined as bilaterally impaired vestibular responses (semicircular canal or otolith responses)
- Able to participate in study procedures including vestibular physiologic testing, balance and gait assessment, neurocognitive testing, and VT or active control
- Able to give informed consent, as further detailed in the Human Subjects section. The investigators anticipate that individuals who are too impaired to provide informed consent would also not be able to effectively participate in VT or active control
- Presence of a caregiver, defined as an individual who spends at least 10 h per week with the patient. The caregiver must be able to participate in study procedures, specifically the text-messaging system. Both the VT and active control involve 8 weeks of once-weekly visits and daily home exercises, and the investigators believe a caregiver would increase the likelihood of successful completion of either therapy

Exclusion Criteria
- Diagnosis of severe AD (CDR ≥3).
- Diagnosis of mild cognitive impairment or diagnosis of non-AD dementia, for example, Parkinson's disease dementia, Dementia with Lewy Bodies, vascular dementia, fronto-temporal dementia, and primary progressive aphasia.
- Deemed unable to participate in study procedures and VT or active control (e.g., patients with significant medical comorbidities, excessive agitation, or use of mobility aids such as a cane or walker).
- Use of daily vestibular suppressant medications, specifically anti-histamines and benzodiazepines, as this can alter the response to VT.
- Lack of availability to participate in 8 weeks of VT or active control.

Ages Eligible for Study
60 Years and older (Adult, Older Adult)

Sexes Eligible for Study
All

Accepts Healthy Volunteers
No

Primary Purpose: Treatment
Allocation: Randomized
Interventional Model: Parallel Assignment
Masking: Triple (Participant Investigator Outcomes Assessor)

Arms and interventions

Participant group/arm	Intervention/treatment
Experimental: vestibular therapy Vestibular therapy (vestibular physical therapy) entails an 8-week course of exercises delivered by a physical therapist designed to improve vestibular function	Behavioral: vestibular physical therapy • Vestibular therapy is a set of exercises delivered by a physical therapist involving head movements. The therapy is delivered over a course of 8 weeks
Active comparator: active control The active control regimen consists of eye movement exercises (e.g., smooth pursuit eye movements) and also general conditioning exercises (e.g., range of motion exercises, lifting light weights with the arms and legs). This regimen is "vestibular neutral" in that head movements which specifically challenge the vestibular system are avoided	Behavioral: active control • Strength and flexibility exercises that do not involve head movements

Primary outcome measures

Outcome measure	Measure description	Time frame
Number of participant falls	Incidence of falls over a 1-year follow-up period	1 year

Sponsor
Johns Hopkins University

Investigators
• Principal Investigator: Yuri Agrawal, MD, Johns Hopkins University

General Publications
No publications available

Treatment

Not Yet Recruiting

United States

Smart Lighting for Nursing Home Residents with Dementia

ClinicalTrials.gov ID NCT05825404

Sponsor Penn State University
Information provided by Ying-Ling Jao RN, PhD, FGSA, Penn State University (Responsible Party)
Last Update Posted 2023-04-24

Study Overview

Brief Summary

This proposed study seeks to develop a smart ambient bright light (SABL) intervention to provide auto-controlled, consistent indoor lighting that incorporates natural daylight. This SABL includes tunable LED lights, photosensors, and controllers. The SABL system has a pre-programmed 24-h control schedule for illuminance settings to mimic the natural bright-dark cycle. It will automatically adjust the lights to accommodate the daylight effect to minimize staff burden and maximize the LI effect. The SABL will be installed in the participants' bedrooms and designated areas in the dining rooms and activity rooms for 4 weeks. Each participant will wear a personal light monitor to measure the lighting dosage each participant receives. This study will address three aims: (1) pilot test the effect of SABL on reducing agitation in persons with ADRD, (2) evaluate the fidelity of the SABL delivery, and (3) evaluate the feasibility of implementing the SABL. The study will be conducted in two NHs in Pennsylvania. For aims 1 and 2, the investigators will use a crossover, cluster randomized control trial (RCT), and will enroll residents with ADRD and agitation. For aim 3, the investigators will use a mixed methods design and will interview NH stakeholders to evaluate the acceptability, feasibility, and appropriateness of the intervention. This is the first study that incorporates daylight in ambient light interventions and the first study that addresses the measurement, feasibility, and fidelity of lighting interventions. Findings will establish evidence-based implementation strategies and the best design for SABL to reduce agitation for persons with ADRD in NHs.

Detailed Description

Up to 90% of people with Alzheimer's disease and related dementias (ADRD) experience at least one behavioral and psychological symptom of dementia (BPSD). Agitation is among the most common and challenging BPSD, especially in nursing home (NH) residents with ADRD. Thus, identifying an effective, nonpharmacological intervention to reduce agitation and other BPSDs is critical. Lighting is important for people with ADRD, especially those living in NHs, as they are not exposed to sufficient daylight. Lighting interventions (LIs) work to regulate suprachiasmatic nuclei, maintain a stable circadian rhythm, and reduce agitation. LIs are not invasive and have minimal adverse effects, making them ideal interventions for persons with ADRD. Evidence has reported that LIs show improvement in agitation and other BPSDs for persons with ADRD. However, LIs have not been widely implemented in "real-world" care settings. Traditional methods using light boxes that required persons with ADRD to sit and keep their eyes oriented toward a bright light led to compliance and workload issues. A more efficient approach to delivering LIs is necessary. Interest has arisen in designing NHs with the capability of providing LIs via ambient LIs. While a few studies have reported positive effects of ambient LIs on agitation, these studies were conducted in settings with window shades closed to minimize daylight. To establish ambient lighting as a feasible and effective intervention, a few fundamental gaps need to be addressed: (1) a feasible implementation approach to ambient LIs and (2) intervention fidelity (ensuring the lighting received by participants meets the targets). This proposed study seeks to develop a smart ambient bright light (SABL) intervention to provide auto-controlled, consistent indoor lighting that incorporates natural daylight. This SABL includes tunable LED lights, photosensors, and controllers. The SABL system has a pre-programmed 24-h control schedule for illuminance settings to mimic the natural bright-dark cycle. It will automatically adjust the lights to accommodate the daylight effect to minimize staff burden and maximize the LI effect. The SABL will be installed in participants' bedrooms and designated areas in the dining rooms and activity rooms for 4 weeks. Each participant will wear a personal light monitor to measure the lighting dosage each participant receives. This study will address three aims: (1) pilot test the effect of SABL on reducing agitation in persons with ADRD, (2) evaluate the fidelity of the SABL delivery, and (3) evaluate the feasibility of implementing the SABL. The study will be conducted in two NHs in Pennsylvania. For aims 1 and 2, the investigators will use a crossover, cluster randomized control trial (RCT), and will enroll residents with ADRD and agitation. For aim 3, the investigators will use a mixed methods design and will interview NH stakeholders to evaluate the acceptability, feasibility, and appropriateness of the intervention. This is the first study that incorporates daylight in ambient light interventions and the first study that addresses the measurement, feasibility, and fidelity of lighting interventions. Findings will establish evidence-based implementation strategies and the best design for SABL to reduce agitation for persons with ADRD in NHs.

Official Title
The Effect of Smart Ambient Bright Light for Nursing Home Residents with
  Alzheimer's Disease and Related Dementias

Alzheimer's Disease and Related Dementias

Intervention/Treatment
- Device: Smart Ambient Bright Light (SABL)
- Other: Control

Other Study ID Numbers
- STUDY00020216

Study Start (Estimated)
2023-04-15

Primary Completion (Estimated)
2023-08-15

Study Completion (Estimated)
2023-12-15

Enrollment (Estimated)
40

Study Type
Interventional

Phase
Not Applicable

Study Contact
Name: Ying-Ling Jao, PhD
Phone Number: 814-865-5634
Email: yuj15@psu.edu

Study Contact Backup
Name: Julian Wang, PhD
Email: Jqw5965@psu.edu
No location data

Inclusion Criteria
- Age ≥55
- English speaking
- Nursing home residency ≥3 months
- Clinical Diagnosis of Alzheimer's Disease and related dementia
- Presence of agitation over the past week

Exclusion Criteria
- Major sleep problems
- Major mental illness
- Severe vision impairment
- Severe acute or terminal illness

Ages Eligible for Study
55 Years and older (Adult, Older Adult)

Sexes Eligible for Study
All

Accepts Healthy Volunteers
No

Primary Purpose: Treatment
Allocation: Randomized
Interventional Model: Crossover Assignment
Masking: Double (Participant Care Provider)

Arms and interventions

Participant group/arm	Intervention/treatment
Experimental: smart ambient bright light The smart ambient bright light (SABL) intervention provides auto-controlled, consistent indoor lighting that incorporates natural daylight	Device: smart ambient bright light (SABL) • The proposed smart ambient bright light (SABL) includes tunable LED lights, photosensors, and controllers. The SABL will provide bright light targeted at 400 lux and CS = 0.3 in participant bedrooms and designated areas such as the dining room and activity room during the day and provide dim light ≤40 lux and CS ≤0.1 in participant bedrooms at night
Sham comparator: control Usual light	Other: control • Usual light

Primary outcome measures

Outcome measure	Measure description	Time frame
Change in the light level: lux at the facility level	Light level (lux) at the facility level will be measured manually on-site	Twice a week for 13 weeks
Change in the light level: CS at the facility level	Light level (CS) at the facility level will be measured manually on-site	Twice a week for 13 weeks
Change in the light level: lux at the individual level	Light level (lux) at the individual level will be measured using a personal light monitor	Weeks 1, 3, 5, 7, 9, 11, and 13
Change in the light level: CS at the individual level	Light level (CS) at the individual level will be measured using a personal light monitor	Weeks 1, 3, 5, 7, 9, 11, and 13
Change in agitation	Agitation will be measured using the Cohen Mansfield Agitation Inventory (CMAI) based on the primary care healthcare workers' (RN, LPN, or CNA) observations over the previous week. The total score ranges from 29 to 203; a higher score indicates a higher agitation level	Weeks 1, 3, 5, 7, 9, 11, and 13
Intervention acceptability	The intervention acceptability of the lighting intervention will be measured based on nursing home stakeholders' perspectives using the Acceptability of Intervention Measure (AIM) and followed up by qualitative interviews. The total score ranges from 12 to 60; a higher score indicates a higher level of acceptability	Week 13
Intervention feasibility	The intervention feasibility of the lighting intervention will be measured based on nursing home stakeholders' perspectives using the Feasibility of Intervention Measure (FIM) and followed up by qualitative interviews. The total score ranges from 9 to 45; a higher score indicates a higher level of feasibility	Week 13
Intervention appropriateness	The intervention appropriateness of the lighting intervention will be measured based on nursing home stakeholders' perspectives using the Intervention Appropriateness Measure (IAM) and followed up by qualitative interviews. The total score ranges from 10 to 50; a higher score indicates a higher level of appropriateness	Week 13

Secondary outcome measures

Outcome measure	Measure description	Time frame
Behavioral and psychological symptoms of dementia (BPSD)	12 BPSDs will be measured, including delusions, hallucinations, dysphoria, euphoria, anxiety, agitation/aggression, apathy, irritability, disinhibition, aberrant motor behaviors, sleep, and appetite. BPSD will be measured using the Neuropsychiatry Inventory-Nursing Home version (NPI-NH). Each behavioral symptom is rated on a 0–3 scale; a higher score indicates a more severe symptom	Weeks 1, 3, 5, 7, 9, 11, and 13
Affect	Six affective states will be measured: contentment, interest, pleasure, anxiety/fear, anger, and sadness, using the Philadelphia Geriatric Center Affect Rating Scale. Each item is rated on a 5-point scale (1–5); a higher score indicates a higher level of effect	Weeks 1, 3, 5, 7, 9, 11, and 13
Adverse effects	Data on intervention-related adverse effects will be collected via inputs from certified nurse assistants (CNAs) using a checklist, which includes deteriorated BPSDs, skin rash, eye irritation, dizziness, nausea, or any other reactions. Each item will be checked as yes or no	Weeks 1, 3, 5, 7, 9, 11, and 13

Sponsor
Penn State University

Investigators
- Principal Investigator: Ying-Ling Jao, PhD, Penn State University

General Publications
- Figueiro MG, Plitnick B, Roohan C, Sahin L, Kalsher M, Rea MS. Effects of a Tailored Lighting Intervention on Sleep Quality, Rest-Activity, Mood, and Behavior in Older Adults With Alzheimer Disease and Related Dementias: A Randomized Clinical Trial. J Clin Sleep Med. 2019 Dec 15;15(12):1757–1767. https://doi.org/10.5664/jcsm.8078. Epub 2019 Nov 8.
- Figueiro MG, Hunter CM, Higgins P, Hornick T, Jones GE, Plitnick B, Brons J, Rea MS. Tailored Lighting Intervention for Persons with Dementia and Caregivers Living at Home. Sleep Health. 2015 Dec 1;1(4):322–330. https://doi.org/10.1016/j.sleh.2015.09.003.
- Jao YL, Wang J, Liao YJ, Parajuli J, Berish D, Boltz M, Van Haitsma K, Wang N, McNally L, Calkins M. Effect of Ambient Bright Light on Behavioral and Psychological Symptoms in People With Dementia: A Systematic Review. Innov Aging. 2022 Mar 24;6(3):igac018. https://doi.org/10.1093/geroni/igac018. eCollection2022.

Treatment

Recruiting

Turkey

Prediction of Effectiveness of rTMS Application in Alzheimer's Patients

ClinicalTrials.gov ID NCT05977088

Sponsor Istanbul Medipol University Hospital
Information provided by Prof. Lutfu Hanoglu, MD, Istanbul Medipol University
    Hospital (Responsible Party)
Last Update Posted 2023-08-04

Brief Summary

Since pharmacological methods are insufficient in the treatment processes of
Alzheimer's disease, nonpharmacological methods such as Transcranial Magnetic
Stimulation (TMS) have started to be tried as a treatment option as in other neurological and psychiatric diseases. Repeated (rTMS) offers a potential treatment path-
way for neurological and psychiatric illnesses. rTMS benefit rate may vary
depending on many factors such as the region where it is applied, the progression,
and the disease degree. This study's aim is to predict the benefit rate to be obtained
from the treatment by using various evaluation parameters before starting rTMS
treatment. Another goal is to develop a personalized TMS treatment protocol based
on the effect of Test Dose TMS on EEG and changes in brain networks that can be
viewed from EEG data generally before and after rTMS treatment. The possible
effects of TMS on Alzheimer's pathophysiology and modification of the disease
process (neuroprotective, anti-inflammatory, and antioxidant) will also be revealed
through blood samples taken from patients before and after treatment. These
approaches also constitute the original value of our study.

Detailed Description

Since pharmacological methods are insufficient in the treatment processes of
Alzheimer's disease, nonpharmacological methods such as Transcranial Magnetic
Stimulation (TMS) have started to be tried as a treatment option as in other neurological and psychiatric diseases. Repeated (rTMS) offers a potential treatment path-way
for neurological and psychiatric illnesses. rTMS benefit rate may vary
depending on many factors such as the region where it is applied, the progression,
and the disease degree. This study's aim is to predict the benefit rate to be obtained
from the treatment by using various evaluation parameters before starting rTMS
treatment. Another goal is to develop a personalized TMS treatment protocol based
on the effect of Test Dose TMS on EEG and change in brain networks that can be
viewed from EEG data generally before and after rTMS treatment. The possible
effects of TMS on Alzheimer's pathophysiology and modification of the disease
process (neuroprotective, anti-inflammatory, and antioxidant) will also be revealed

through blood samples taken from patients before and after treatment. These approaches also constitute the original value of our study.

In our project, 20 people will be included in the study and control groups, and electroencephalography (EEG) and TMS will be used together in the study. Before rTMS treatment, resting EEG data will be taken for 5 min, eyes open and closed. After then, Test Dose TMS of 150 beats at 20 Hz will be applied to the left dorsolateral prefrontal cortex. Immediately after this Test Dose rTMS, the patient's resting state EEG data will be taken again. At the end of all these procedures, rTMS treatment will be started, which will take 5 days. The treatment will consist of 2 sessions per day with a 20 Hz stimulating protocol, 1500 beats to right-left DLPFC, and totally 3000 beats. EEG recordings will be taken again from all patients 1 week after the treatment.

Changes in the cognitive functions of Alzheimer's patients will be made through the neuropsychometric test battery taken before and after rTMS. With the analysis of neuropsychometric data, the study group will be divided into two subgroups that benefit from TMS and those who do not, the effect of Test Dose TMS on EEG will be investigated, the algorithm that predicts individuals who will benefit from TMS through pre-TMS EEG data and Test Dose TMS-EEG data will be investigated and the effect of TMS treatment on EEG will be investigated. Therefore, the prediction algorithm will open the door to personalized treatment protocol. In addition, EEG data obtained before and after TMS will be compared with power spectrum, coherence, functional connectivity, and graph methods in both the study and control groups, and information about the electrophysiological effects of TMS will be obtained.

Blood samples of the patients before and after rTMS will be taken and the changes in the metabolites given below will be compared: brain-derived neurotrophic factor, glial-based neurotrophic factor, total oxidant level, total antioxidant level, oxidative stress index, total thiol, native thiol, disulfide, exosome, inflammation biomarkers (interleukin 1 beta, interleukin 6, tumor necrosis alpha, interferon gamma, and nuclear factor kappa ß), Albumin Globulin ratio, Omega 6 and Omega 3. Thus, rTMS has possible neuroprotective, anti-inflammatory, and antioxidant effects, consequently modifying the disease process. Additional information will be obtained about.

Within the scope of the project, a workshop, sharing of study results in national-international congresses, a patent application originating from algorithm production, production of three graduate students' thesis, and at least three scientific articles will be produced. In addition, the investigators anticipate that TMS prevalence will increase during the treatment process of Alzheimer's patients, and the socio-economic burden.

Official Title

Prediction of Cognitive, Neurotrophic, Anti-Inflammatory, and Antioxidant Effectiveness of rTMS Application in Alzheimer's Patients by Combination of Test-Dose TMS and EEG

Conditions
Alzheimer Disease

Intervention/Treatment
• Device: Repetitive Transcranial Magnetic Stimulation

Other Study ID Numbers
• 221S749

Study Start (Actual)
2022-02-16

Primary Completion (Estimated)
2025-05-15

Study Completion (Estimated)
2025-05-15

Enrollment (Estimated)
40

Study Type
Interventional

Phase
Not Applicable

Study Contact
Name: Lutfu Hanoglu, Prof. DR. MD
Phone Number: +90444 8544
Email: lhanoglu@kure.com.tr

Study Contact Backup
Name: Cennet Sena Parlatan, PhD Cand
Phone Number: 05077799164
Email: cennetsenaparlatan@gmail.com
Turkey

Istanbul, Turkey, 34214
Recruiting
Medipol University Hospital

Contact
Lutfu Hanoglu, MD, PhD
0090 212460 70 30 lhanoglu@kure.com.tr

Principal Investigator
Lutfu Hanoglu, MD, PhD

Inclusion Criteria
- Have been diagnosed with clinical Alzheimer's Disease in accordance with the NINCDS-ADRDA diagnostic criteria
- >55 years old
- Clinical Dementia Rating Scale (CDR) score in the 1–2 range
- Not having any other disease that affects their cognitive functions
- Volunteer to participate in the study

Exclusion Criteria
- Participant or relative does not give consent
- The patient's inability to participate in the entire study procedure (e.g., living in another city)
- The patient's history of head trauma with alcohol/substance abuse
- Presence of severe stroke and other neurological sequelae disease in the participant
- Presence of a metal implant on the head or having a pacemaker and contraindications for other TMS applications During the study or 1 month before, having/been receiving/receiving an investigational drug targeting Alzheimer's disease or neuromodulation treatment such as tDCS and TMS, other than standard treatment for AD symptom control such as acetylcholine esterase and memantine, with the potential to affect the study

Ages Eligible for Study
- 55 Years and older (Adult, Older Adult)

Sexes Eligible for Study
- All

Accepts Healthy Volunteers
- No

Design Details
- Primary Purpose: Diagnostic
Allocation: Randomized
Interventional Model: Parallel Assignment
Masking: Single (Participant)

Arms and interventions

Participant group/arm	Intervention/treatment

Experimental: interventional
Power Mag TMS device will be used throughout the study, and the excitations will be made with the help of an 8 shaped coil (diameter: 70 mm) with internal cooling. The right-left DLPFC, which is the application area, will be determined with the help of the primary motor hand area and the 10/20 EEG system
Patients will be given two stimulations (pulse duration = 3.5 s, interval between beats = 45 s) consisting of only 75 beats, 100% of the cap threshold value compatible with the magnetic field TMS determined just before the rTMS routine application, and a total of 150 pulses of Test Dose TMS will be applied. A resting state EEG (eyes open-closed) will be taken immediately after (max. 2 min later) in the Faraday cage
	Device: repetitive transcranial magnetic stimulation
	• Power Mag TMS device will be used throughout the study, and the excitations will be made with the help of an 8 shaped coil (diameter: 70 mm) with internal cooling. The right-left DLPFC, which is the application area, will be determined with the help of the primary motor hand area and the 10/20 EEG system
	   Patients will be given two stimulations (pulse duration = 3.5 s, interval between beats = 45 s) consisting of only 75 beats, 100% of the cap threshold value compatible with the magnetic field TMS determined just before the rTMS routine application, and a total of 150 pulses of Test Dose TMS will be applied. A resting state EEG (eyes open-closed) will be taken immediately after (max. 2 min later) in the Faraday cage. The same procedures will be done with the sham coil in the control group
	• Other Names:
	  – Electroencephalography

Sham comparator: sham
The same treatment procedures will be applied to the control group with a sham coil
	Device: repetitive transcranial magnetic stimulation
	• Power Mag TMS device will be used throughout the study, and the excitations will be made with the help of an 8 shaped coil (diameter: 70 mm) with internal cooling. The right-left DLPFC, which is the application area, will be determined with the help of the primary motor hand area and the 10/20 EEG system
	   Patients will be given two stimulations (pulse duration = 3.5 s, interval between beats = 45 s) consisting of only 75 beats, 100% of the cap threshold value compatible with the magnetic field TMS determined just before the rTMS routine application, and a total of 150 pulses of Test Dose TMS will be applied. A resting state EEG (eyes open-closed) will be taken immediately after (max. 2 min later) in the Faraday cage. The same procedures will be done with the sham coil in the control group
	• Other Names:
	  – Electroencephalography

Primary outcome measures

Outcome measure	Measure description	Time frame
The mini mental state examination	Cognitive neuropsychological test score	Changes before treatment and 1 month after treatment
Neuropsychiatric inventory	Cognitive neuropsychological test score	Changes before treatment and 1 month after treatment
Alzheimer's Disease Assessment Scale	Cognitive neuropsychological test score	Changes before treatment and 1 month after treatment
ADSL	Cognitive neuropsychological test score	Changes before treatment and 1 month after treatment
Geriatric Depression Scale	Cognitive neuropsychological test score	Changes before treatment and 1 month after treatment

Secondary outcome measures

Outcome measure	Measure description	Time frame
Blood samples ELISA analyses	BDNF: measured spectrophotometrically with commercially purchased ELISA kits. GDNF: measured spectrophotometrically with commercially purchased ELISA kits. Exosome: measured spectrophotometrically with commercially available ELISA kits Anti-inflammatory cytokines: IL-1β, IL-6, TNF-α, IFNy, NF-kβ values will be measured spectrophotometrically with commercially purchased ELISA kits	Changes before treatment and 1 month after treatment
Blood samples analyses	OSI:TOS and TAS will be measured by photometric methods. OSI will be found by mathematical calculation. Total thiol and native thiol concentrations are measured spectrophotometrically in separate solutions prepared for the determination of the thiol-disulfite ratio, which is another indicator of oxidative stress, and the amount of disulfide is determined according to the mathematical ratio between them Albumin globulin ratio: measured by electrophoresis method and albumin globulin ratio will be determined Omega 6/3 levels: determined by commercially purchased lipid mediators	Changes before treatment and 1 month after treatment
Inflammatory biomarker analyses	Inflammatory parameters IL-1β, IL-6, and TNF-α will be measured IL-1β, IL-6, and TNF-α levels will be measured photometrically with commercially available ELISA kits	Changes before treatment and 1 month after treatment

Outcome measure	Measure description	Time frame
Oxidative stress biomarker analyses	TAS, TOS, TT, and NT levels of oxidative stress parameters in blood samples taken from AD patients will be measured. TAS, TOS, TT, and NT levels of blood samples taken will be measured by photometric method with kits to be purchased commercially. The oxidative stress index (OSI) will be found as TOS/TAS, and the amount of dynamic disulfide bonds will be found by determining half of the difference between the TT and NT groups	Changes before treatment and 1 month after treatment
Evaluation of fatty acid profile analysis with GC-MS	Fatty acids comprising more than 95% of the fatty acids detectable in plasma will be measured Tetradecanoic acid, 9(Z)-Tetradecenoic acid, Hexadecanoic acid, 9(Z)-Hexadecenoic acid, 9(E)-Hexadecenoic acid, Octadecanoic acid, 9(Z)-Octadecenoic acid, Methyl 9(E)-Octadecenoate, 11(Z)-Octadecenoic acid, Methyl 11(E)-Octadecenoate, Methyl 6(Z)-Octadecenoate, 9(Z),12(Z)-Octadecadienoic acid, 9(E),12(E)-Octadecadienoic acid, 9(Z),12(Z),15(Z)-Octadecatrienoic acid, 6(Z),9(Z),12(Z)-Octadecatrienoic acid, Eicosanoic acid, 8(Z),11(Z),14(Z)-Eicosatrienoic acid, 5(Z),8(Z),11(Z),14(Z)-Eicosatetraenoic acid, 11(Z)-Eicosenoic acid, 11(Z),14(Z)-Eicosadienoic acid, 5(Z),8(Z),11(Z),14(Z),17(Z)-Eicosapentaenoic acid, Docosanoic acid, 13(Z)-Docosenoic acid, 4(Z),7(Z),10(Z),13(Z),16(Z),19(Z)-Docosahexaenoic acid, 7(Z),10(Z),13(Z),16(Z)-Docosatetraenoic acid, 7(Z),10(Z),13(Z),16(Z),19(Z)-Docosapentaenoic acid, 4(Z),7(Z),10(Z),13(Z),16(Z)-Docosapentaenoic acid, Tetracosanoic acid, and 15(Z)-Tetracosenoic acid	Changes before treatment and 1 month after treatment

Outcome measure	Measure description	Time frame
Metabolomics analysis by liquid chromatography-mass spectrometer/mass spectrometer (LC-MS/MS)	The 41 amino acids to look for by LC-MS/MS are: 1. 1-Methylhistidine 2. 2-Aminoadipic acid 3. 3-Aminoisobutyric acid 4. 3-Methylhistidine 5. 4-Hydroxyproline 6. 5-Hydroxylysine 7. Alanine 8. Alloisoleucine 9. Anserine 10. Arginine 11. Argininosuccinic acid 12. Asparagine 13. β-Alanine 14. Carnosine 15. Citrulline 16. Cystine 17. Cystathionine 18. Ethanolamine 19. Gamma-aminobutyric acid 20. Glutamine 21. Glutamic acid 22. Histidine 23. Homocitrulline 24. Isoleucine 25. Leucine 26. Lysine 27. Methionine 28. Norvaline 29. *O*-Phosphorylethanolamine 30. *O*-Phosphoserine 31. Ornithine 32. Phenylanalanine 33. Proline 34. Sarcosine 35. Serine 36. Taurine 37. Threonine 38. Trans-4-hydroxyproline 39. Tryptophan 40. Tyrosine 41. Valine	Changes before treatment and 1 month after treatment

Outcome measure	Measure description	Time frame
EEG power spectrum analysis	EEG data will be separated into 1-s epochs after they are cleared of noise. Power spectrums of these data will be obtained in the delta, theta, alpha, beta, and gamma frequency bands. Each epoch will be analyzed by Fast Fourier Transform (FFT, Fast Fourier Transform) with 10% Hanning window, then power spectrum analysis will be performed, giving the frequency values for each electrode by averaging all FFTs. Maximum peaks will be determined in the delta (0.5–3.5 Hz), theta (4–7 Hz), alpha (8–13 Hz), beta (15–28 Hz), and gamma (28–48 Hz) frequency bands. These values will be used in statistical analysis for each person and electrode	Changes before treatment and 1 month after treatment
EEG coherence analysis	Coherence measurements at delta, theta, alpha, beta, and gamma frequencies can be analyzed for either intra-hemispheric electrode connections or inter-hemispheric electrode connections. Coherence values take values between 0 and −1. Values close to 0 indicate that there is no connection at the determined frequency between the two calculated electrode regions, while values close to 1 indicate a high coupling between the two electrode regions. Coherence values will be calculated with the Brain Vision Analyzer program using the formula below. The data obtained during memory and visualization will be separated into 1-s epochs after they are cleared of noise. Power spectrums of these data will be obtained in the delta, theta, alpha, beta, and gamma frequency bands. Each epoch will be analyzed by Fast Fourier Transform with 10% Hanning window. Then, these data will be calculated for all possible electrode pairs using the brain vision analysis program with the formula given below	Changes before treatment and 1 month after treatment

Outcome measure	Measure description	Time frame
EEG functional connectivity analysis	eLORETA software will be used for functional connectivity analysis. sLORETA/eLORETA is an online free software developed by Roberto Pascual-Marqui and his team (http://www.uzh.ch/keyinst/loreta.htm). eLORETA is an algorithm developed to solve the inverse problem and it does not contain localization bias even in the presence of noise. In this software, resting state data with eyes closed, separated into 2 s epochs, whose artifacts are cleaned by preprocessing, will be used. The relevant areas to be analyzed in the cortical plane and the relevant frequency band gaps will be determined. The time series containing the eLORETA current source density obtained from these areas will be calculated and a "lagged linear coherence" matrix will be created to be applied in graph theory. "Lagged linear coherence" will give correct physiological connectivity unaffected by volume conduction and low spatial resolution	Changes before treatment and 1 month after treatment
EEG analysis by machine learning	The machine learning method was created based on the current experimental design and the planned number of patients. After the data are cleared and ready for analysis, the differences in the EEG signals of the patients who benefited from rTMS after the Test Dose TMS from the EEG signals after the Test Dose TMS of the patients who did not benefit will be revealed by a classification method. For this purpose, it is planned to implement the Support Vector Machines (SVM) method. The DVM method is the most suitable for our data and the project purpose among the machine learning methods with its high classification success in large-sized data that is difficult to parse	Changes before treatment and 1 month after treatment

Sponsor

Istanbul Medipol University Hospital

Collaborators

- Bezmialem Vakif University
- Saglik Bilimleri Universitesi

Investigators

- Principal Investigator: Lutfu Hanoglu, Prof. DR. MD, Medipol University

General Publications

No publications available

Index